A Recipe for Hope

HOW WE FOUGHT CANCER WITH FAMILY, FRIENDS, FAITH, AND FOOD

JEFFERY WEAVER

Brea, California
2016

A Recipe for Hope: How We Fought Cancer with Family, Friends, Faith, and Food

Printed in the United States of America

First Printing, 2016

Jeffery Weaver
Brea, California

www.jefferyweaver.com

Edited and designed by The Artful Editor
www.artfuleditor.com
Cover design by Marija Vilotijevic
Interior design by Catherine Murray

ISBN 978-0-9982841-0-1 (hardcover)
ISBN 978-0-9982841-2-5 (paperback)

Dedication

To my wife, Susan, who has shown me how to lead a better life, and shown us all how to be tough, gracious, and kind.

Also, to every cancer patient who faces the uncertainty that comes with a cancer diagnosis. Susan would say, "Just don't give up." I would add, keep the faith because there is always hope.

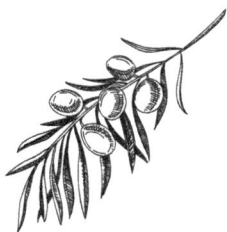

Contents

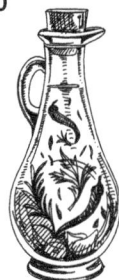

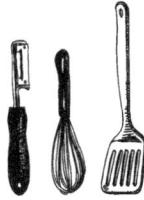

Foreword

Dr. Simon Davies

THE CIA (Central Intelligence Agency) ranks the United States of America among other countries at number 51 in longevity. Despite being a superpower, and despite the billions of dollars spent on our healthcare system, we are systematically poisoning ourselves to early deaths with foods, food additives, pesticides, and many of the drugs we put into our bodies. Why is this self-inflicted threat to our national security being tolerated, if not sanctioned? Profit margin has a great influence, so the agribusiness, chemicalized food, pharmaceutical, and medical conglomerates dictate how food is produced, promoted, and consumed. And then an elaborate system of medications, prescriptions, and medical procedures deals with the consequences. Attempts to protect the consumer are systematically undermined by powerful interest groups and their political lackeys. A classic example of this is the ongoing battle to prevent the labeling—not the removal—of food items containing genetically modified organisms (GMOs).

Cancer is so prevalent, and devastating, in American society, that billions of dollars are spent on research in an attempt to find a cure. Unfortunately, although progress has been made, the most frequently used therapies, chemotherapy and radiation, are often ineffective and in many cases have been found to hasten or cause death in late-stage patients. With this Damoclean sword hanging over us, what path should we take to prevent and cure this devastating disease? People need to be aware that they have a choice between utilizing their own body or relying solely upon external interventions.

Branches of cancer research focus efforts on understanding the reason why typically healthy cells mutate, which can result in rampant cell growth, leading to possible tumors and cancer. Potential triggers to this cellular rebranding include many of the components of our hectic and unbalanced lifestyles. The accumulation of toxins in our tissues from the contaminated air and water and the consumption of food grown with pesticides and insecticides, of factory-farmed animals raised on antibiotics and growth hormones, and of chemicalized food laced with genetically modified and unpronounceable ingredients, preservatives, and colorings raises the question: What chance do our cells have against this constant alien bombardment? Are the cellular mutations and the resultant diseases any surprise?

In my many years of working with athletes, I have emphasized balanced nutrition because it is of paramount importance. The body must be optimally fueled to achieve peak performance. The diet must work in harmony with the body's requirements. Anti-inflammatory foods, such as those containing high levels of omega-3 fatty acids, can play a significant role in preventing injuries, reducing recovery time, and improving overall health. Athletes also benefit from increased circulation, which provides a greater supply of nutrients and oxygen to the cells. Foods such as ginger, cayenne pepper, citrus, and goji berries all have significant circulatory effects. Although the general population perhaps does not require such a detailed, event-specific level of nutrition precision, they can still gain greatly by eating foods that increase their overall level of health, their resistance to disease, their recuperative ability, and ultimately their longevity.

Jeff Weaver's book makes a powerful contribution in this scenario. Powerful not because the outcome was lifesaving—which is brilliant and amazing in itself—but because the remedy involves utilizing the body's own recuperative abilities and avoiding all the side effects of traditional cancer treatments. We see a genuinely honest and heartfelt attempt to incorporate a holistic and person-centered approach to dealing with a terminal case of cancer. This book is a road map, a template, that any individual who feels abandoned by "Western medicine" can follow. No claims are made that the information in this book will work for everyone. Details are provided of what worked so successfully for Jeff and his wife, Susan. The body has incredible resilience and amazing powers of recuperation and recovery. To battle cancer, we need to supply it with the nutrients it requires, maximizing its combat capacity, mobilizing all its resources, giving it a fighting chance!

Simon Davies, PhD
Professor, Kinesiology and Health
Irvine Valley College

Dr. Simon Davies has taught health and nutrition at the University of Greenwich, London; University of California, Davis; and Albion College, Michigan. Additionally, he has taught classes in sport psychology and has coached varsity soccer. Dr. Davies has been a vegetarian for twenty-five years and a vegan for fifteen years.

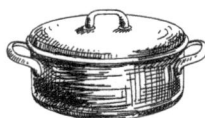

Introduction

I WISH I hadn't written this book. But I had to write this book because my wife, Susan, was diagnosed with breast cancer. That in itself doesn't make her special—she is just one of 14.1 million people who were diagnosed with cancer in 2012, or, to put it another way, every day in that year, 22,000 people found out they too had cancer. Sadly, 8.2 million people died from cancer in 2012. What makes Susan special is how she fought her deadly disease.

In 2009, I had gone back to college to advance my career in the field of economics. I was required to retake academic writing classes. I protested, but that didn't work. But as I went through the different courses I met a couple of professors who saw something in me and encouraged me to pursue writing. Later, after I completed the required courses, I enrolled in a few creative writing classes.

When Susan was first diagnosed with cancer, I asked Lisa Alvarez, one of my creative writing professors, about doing a blog to make it easier to keep family and friends up-to-date on my wife's medical condition and how she was holding up. Professor Alvarez thought a blog was a great idea and helped me get started. After I began researching cancer and cancer treatments, the purpose of the blog quickly changed. Thousands of studies on cancer and cancer treatments exist, and I even ran across a few on the link between diet and cancer. The problem was that I knew there was an agenda behind many of the studies done on certain foods because billions of dollars are on the line for many agribusinesses. I also found that good information was scattered across many different media that most people don't have the time or know-how to find. However, this was one of the biggest challenges of my life—I *had* to make the time, and, fortunately, because of my profession, I had access to research that most people don't. As one of the managing directors of Premier Capital Partners, a research and investment firm that represents publicly traded companies, one of my jobs was to research up-and-coming companies that offered innovative products or services. So, I made it a point to look for companies involved in the newest cancer studies and the latest drug trials. Then, I expanded the scope of my research to how foods, exercise, and mental attitudes could help fight cancer.

As I gathered all the research papers from the multitude of studies being conducted around the world, it dawned on me that, with all the information I had, I might really be able to help Susan extend her life or even win her fight. It was kind of like doing a jigsaw puzzle because I had to figure out how to put all these different pieces together.

I think most husbands view themselves as problem solvers. But when you are told your wife has only three to five years to live and that her cancer is incurable, you wonder, how can I solve that? Fortunately for me, the puzzle pieces quickly started to fall into place. I could see the picture more clearly as each bit came together: I knew I couldn't do anything medically other than to try to understand the drugs Susan was treated with and how they would affect her then and in the future. But when it came to food and lifestyle, there was plenty I could do to help Susan. Like that old saying "the straw that broke the camel's back," I figured that's exactly what we would do—throw every straw we could find on the back of her cancer and pray that it would break, that all that straw would weigh enough to tip the scales in her favor.

I talked to Susan about this. She was a little skeptical at first, but given what she had been told by her doctors, she was willing to try.

The more research and reading I did, the more it became apparent that lifestyle and diet play huge parts in our ability to fight disease. In some cases, these are as important as drugs and medicine.

At first I used what I found to help only Susan. But my efforts soon morphed into helping others as I began posting my findings on the blog. Nearly every person I talked to had a close friend or family member who had cancer or who had had cancer. With the blog, in the last few years I've told hundreds of people about Susan's amazing journey and her incredible will to win the fight. Almost everyone who has heard her story was truly moved, and often moved to tears. Many of them told me I should write a book about her.

I thought, *Why not?* That way I could share what I had learned, and doing so might help others avoid ever having to go through the life-and-death struggle that accompanies a cancer diagnosis.

So, here we are, and that blog is the genesis of this book. I decided to use the journal format of the blog in order to preserve the real-time telling of Susan's journey. It's a sort of a road map others can use to follow the story of the bravest woman I know as she journeyed from hopelessness to hope. You can use it to learn what you can do to fight or prevent cancer. May you be as awed as I was at the account of how this one woman fought cancer one step at a time, one day at a time, and one bite at a time.

(Cancer statistics are from the International Agency for Research on Cancer/ World Health Organization, 2012.)

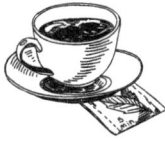

PART I

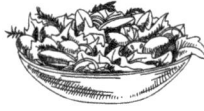

Susan's Story

I DON'T know the exact date Susan's trouble started, but I know who told us about it.

Although I hadn't noticed anything different, in the last months of winter in 2011 Susan commented several times about Jessica's odd behavior: her worried expressions, her clinginess, her agitation. Susan asked Jessica what was bothering her and why she was acting so distressed. Her behavior was puzzling.

So, who is Jessica? She's not our daughter, but she is a family member. Jessica Jazz is our red tricolored Australian shepherd. She is the smartest dog I have ever met and has the best sense of smell of any dog I've been around. Susan and Jessie have a special connection.

One day Susan said, "I think Jessie is trying to tell me something is wrong." I had learned to listen to Susan about her intuitions, so I asked her what Jessie was trying to say. She said she didn't really know, but Jessica had been following her around and would stand in her way if she tried to leave the house. Jessica went so far as to follow Susan into the bathroom, where she became even more distressed, and pushed her nose in places it really didn't belong. She had never done that before.

Then I started noticing it, too. Susan would sit down, and Jessie would lie on Susan's feet and wrap her legs around Susan's, as if she was holding on to her. She literally wouldn't let Susan out of sight. Everywhere Susan went, Jessie went.

Then I remembered something Susan had said to me earlier that summer. We had been talking about some personal problem we were having when Susan abruptly said, "Well, it doesn't matter because I probably won't be around anyway." I was surprised and asked what she meant. She couldn't or wouldn't tell me, so I let it go, but I did not forget her words. They really bothered me.

Jessie's odd behavior continued, and she became even more clingy. Then, on February 6, 2012, Susan told me she felt a lump in her breast. We didn't panic because this wasn't the first time she had felt lumps. A few years earlier she had discovered a couple of lumps in a self-examination and had them biopsied. Luckily, the test came back negative, and Susan was told she had dense breasts and lumps were fairly common in women who had dense breast tissue. This time, we thought it prudent to call her doctor. He made the referral and we got an appointment scheduled for two days later with Dr. Julio Vaquerano, a surgical oncologist at Kaiser Permanente, who we have our health plan with.

Susan and I went in together, and he examined her. Afterward, we sat down with him and he too told us that because she had dense breasts lumps were common. He didn't think these were cancerous, so he said not to worry. He ordered a mammogram, and it was done on February 15. The results showed enough information that biopsies were scheduled.

On February 21, we got a message that her oncologist had been changed because Dr. Vaquerano was an emergency doctor. The next day, Susan had biopsies taken on two lumps in the left breast.

The next few days were stressful for both of us, but more so for Susan. We waited forever for the results. I told Susan that the interminable wait was actually good news because if something was wrong she would hear from the doctor sooner rather than later. I felt confident that everything was going to be okay because Susan hadn't been losing weight or feeling any unusual pain, typical symptoms of cancer. But a nagging voice in the back of my head kept repeating Susan's words from last summer: "I probably won't be around anyway."

I could see that Susan was overwhelmed by all this and was really scared. But she went about her life, and her job became a sanctuary of sorts, because it took her mind off things.

On Monday, February 27, Susan went to work in Laguna Hills at Macy's, where she was the merchandising lead. She said she was sitting in the lunchroom when she got a call from Kaiser. She was alone, so she answered. A nurse asked if Susan could talk. When Susan said yes, the nurse told her that the biopsy results were positive and that Susan had breast cancer. Susan said she was able to stay calm for a minute. Then, the nurse told her that they had also found a lump in her right breast and one and possibly more lymph nodes in her left armpit that needed to be biopsied as well. She told Susan that she needed to come in the next day and meet with Craig Emmons, a physician's assistant, who would fill her in on what would happen going forward. The nurse said the new biopsies were scheduled for the twenty-ninth. When she heard that, Susan said her heart started to pound and she felt like she would vomit.

She said she was so shook up she called her boss, Jesus, who was out to lunch.

Jesus and Susan had always been really close, and he knew something was drastically wrong when she told him she had to go home. He asked her to please wait a couple minutes until he got there.

When he walked into his office, he found Susan sitting in silence and shaking all over. I don't know about others, but only a couple times in my life have I been so frightened that it caused me to shake uncontrollably—and I have never seen Susan react this way. She said that Jesus asked her what was wrong, and she told him she just found out she had cancer.

Before he let her leave work, Jesus told her he had had other friends who had battled cancer. He said, "Whatever you do, just don't give up."

That night at home we called Ann and Martin, Susan's folks, and then mine to tell them. I called our twenty-four-year-old daughter, Nicole, and told her. Nicki is really close to her mom, and this was a tough conversation. She freaked out on the phone and started to cry uncontrollably. When our son, Josh, who is twenty-five and lives at home with us, got in from work, we talked to him. Josh is very good at hiding his feelings. He acts tough, but I know he was really upset. Later that evening Susan made a call to a very special young friend of hers, Francesca. That was the first time I saw her cry. We barely slept that night because the reality of her diagnosis started to hit us.

Susan went to work for half a day on the twenty-eighth and told her close friend and coworker, Martha, and the store manager, Maria. But she didn't tell her other coworkers. When she left Macy's that afternoon, no one knew Susan wouldn't be back.

Later that afternoon at three o'clock, we met with Craig Emmons at the Kaiser Permanente medical offices on Sand Canyon in Irvine. Craig was doing all the scheduling and setting up all the appointments. He sat with us, explaining everything and telling us what to expect, but most importantly, he let us know that Susan would be in excellent hands and to try not to worry. Right, I thought. He then told us that Susan had been selected for Kaiser's Multi-Dimensional Team. She would have more testing than most, and a team of doctors would review her case and decide together what course of action to take. That made us feel pretty good, but it also raised alarms. Why her?

Craig was wonderful, and he really made us feel like he was looking out for Susan.

On the twenty-ninth, Susan went in for the additional biopsies. She told me that she watched the screen as the doctor inserted the biopsy needle. She could see the lump they had biopsied years before because of a metal marker left in it to identify it. She said that lump looked round with smooth edges. Then she saw the lump they had biopsied a couple days ago, and it was big and had really uneven edges. She told me it was then she knew this might be big trouble.

The next day, Thursday, March 1, Susan, Nicole, and I met with the doctors who were part of the Multi-Dimensional Team. First, we saw Dr. Luby, the surgeon, a really nice lady. She told us that

Susan would have a double mastectomy and that the tumor in her left breast was the most worrisome because it was large and had already grown into the chest wall, which made it dangerous. The second tumor in the left breast was small, so the surgeon wasn't too worried about it, and the tumors in the right breast were also small. They were well inside the breast, so Dr. Luby was confident she should be able to remove all the cancerous cells.

Then we talked to Dr. Iyer, the plastic surgeon who would do reconstructive surgery should Susan want it. He explained the various ways it could be done. Radiation therapy was required before reconstruction to ensure all the cancerous cells that might be left behind after the mastectomy were killed. Because of where the large tumor was located and how far it had grown into the chest wall, he couldn't do reconstruction in the same surgery as the mastectomy because it could jeopardize how effective the radiation was later. Implants could shield any leftover cancer cells from the radiation. He said Susan would have to wait a few months after the mastectomy before he could do the reconstructive surgery, so there was plenty of time for her to decide what she wanted to do. This news made me uncomfortable. I was worried about the risk of performing another surgery so long after Susan had healed from the mastectomy. Susan, on the other hand, was pretty set on having the reconstruction done.

Next we saw Dr. Hoffman from genetics. He told us they would do a blood test that uses DNA analysis to identify harmful mutations in either one of two breast cancer susceptibility genes, *BRCA1* and *BRCA2*. Women who inherit the mutations in their genes are at much higher risk for breast cancer and ovarian cancer than women who do not. He looked pointedly at us while saying that it would be good to know whether Susan had the mutations because, if so, Nicole might also have inherited them. I looked over at Nicole. Her expression immediately changed from that of a daughter standing by her mom to a woman who may have inherited a huge worry. At the very least, the next few days were going to be a lot different for her than she had ever imagined.

At last we were escorted into a meeting room where we were introduced to Susan's oncologist, Dr. Asuncion. We sat at a big round table. I was on Dr. Asuncion's immediate right, Susan was across from her, and Nicole sat next to Susan. I was struck by how young Dr. Asuncion looked, but after listening to her I felt like she was the right oncologist for Susan. She had an easy, gentle way about her. She explained everything thoroughly. Her voice was soft and soothing. As she talked to us, a nurse knocked and came into the room immediately. She handed Dr. Asuncion a piece of paper folded in half. The doctor opened the page and read. Total silence descended on the room. Dr. Asuncion kind of gasped and then put her hand to her mouth. I looked at her intently, thinking, *Oh, shit . . . this isn't good*. I looked at Susan and over at Nicole. We all turned to the doctor and waited for her to speak.

Finally, after what felt like ten minutes, Dr. Asuncion looked up from the paper and at Susan. Her manner was very serious and subdued. Indicating the paper, she said that it was the results of the latest biopsies. She waited for a minute, and then she said, "There is no other way to say this, but the biopsies are positive and you have two separate cancers. This is rare. I am so sorry."

I looked over at Susan and all the color was gone from her face. I reached over and took her hand. Neither of us said anything, but I could feel her shaking, and she squeezed my hand hard. I can't remember whether Nicole said anything. Then Dr. Asuncion's voice cut through all the confusion and panic racing around in my mind. Her calming voice brought me back to the moment. She told us this was bad, but it could have been worse; however, it didn't look like the cancers had spread. Nevertheless, she ordered additional testing to confirm. We said our goodbyes and headed for the car. All three of us were stunned. My head was spinning. We had gotten a ton of information, but it was the bombshell that Susan had two separate cancers that was hard for me to digest.

On the way home I realized we were in for a long, tough fight with an uncertain outcome. I knew a lot about combatting cancer and what Susan was facing because I had battled metastatic cancer myself just a few years earlier. I wondered why we had to go through this again. What had we done to deserve this? For the past several years, life had been hard because we had lost everything in the dot-com crash. Plus, when I was diagnosed with cancer we didn't have health insurance, so we had to pay all the medical expenses for my treatments out of pocket. Then came a succession of jobs at companies that went out of business, leaving me with lots of bounced paychecks if they had bothered to pay me at all. To top it off, Susan's cancer could not have come at a worse time for us financially because my current job was in a dying industry and my income was nearly nonexistent at times. I had taken a big financial risk when I went back to college a couple years earlier, hoping to improve my chances and future. But the most important thing at the moment was Susan's health. I had to figure out how best to help her and get us back on track financially.

After dinner we sat down and talked about all this and decided that the best thing we could do is just get through this day and then worry about the next one, and then the one after that.

I sat in my chair, my mind going a thousand miles an hour. Mick, my Aussie, was at my feet. He is a very happy dog, and as long as he is with his people and they aren't upset with him, then all is right in his world. I glanced over at Susan. Jessie was lying down with her legs wrapped tightly around Susan's ankles and her head resting against Susan's shin. All was not right in her world. Something was terribly wrong with her best friend.

On Saturday, March 2, we went to the infusion center at the hospital and met with the oncology team. They gave us the grand tour of the place. We walked down the central hall, and all the small side rooms were filled with cancer patients sitting in big leather chairs. Some were bald, and many wore scarves or hats to hide the effects of chemo treatments or to stay warm. Next to each chair was a tall metal stand with clear plastic bags hanging from the horizontal bar at the top. The bags of toxic drugs had tubes coming out of the bottom that ran down to the patients' arms, where white gauze bandages partially hid large-gauge needles stuck in the skin. The nurse explained how the process went and she introduced us to the other nurses. Everyone seemed nice and surprisingly upbeat considering they were surrounded by cancer patients, many of whom were fighting for their lives. Our tour guide took us to a room and gave a detailed explanation of the do's and don'ts while Susan was taking chemotherapy treatments. She warned that Susan should never eat raw foods because they are a prime source of bacteria, salmonella, and listeria and one of the biggest risks she'd face was infection. Susan's white blood cell count was going to be low, and her immune system would be weakened tremendously by the drugs. Then she showed a video on chemotherapy treatments. It was depressing and frankly kind of bothered us because it warned of all the side effects from the chemo drugs, how sick Susan was going to get, and the potential of contracting life-threatening illnesses.

When the video was over, the nurse brought in several blankets that volunteers had made and asked Susan to pick one to keep herself warm while she was getting her treatments. Susan chose a black one with lots of pink hearts. Then the nurse gave us the schedule for Susan's chemo treatments. The first one was on the fifth, two days away. Before Susan could start her treatments she had to go see a dentist to make sure her teeth were good and had no problems that would cause an infection. She also had to get a MUGA test (MUGA stands for *multigated acquisition* and is a type of scan that detects the functioning of the lower chambers of the heart) to see whether her heart was strong enough to hold up under the chemo drug she would be taking. That scared the crap out of both of us. How bad was this stuff anyway?

We didn't know what would happen next. That would depend on the results of the scans and other tests. Susan had a very good personal support team in her family and her many friends. Another thing Susan had going for her was her spirit and will. Even though she faced an unknown future, she was more concerned about how her family was doing rather than about what she confronted. I didn't know how she did this or what she really felt behind the brave front she put on.

Right then, all I hoped for was that she stayed strong. I prayed that God would help us and guide us down the new road we were about to travel.

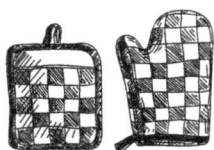

And Now We Fight

Adventures (Part I)

By Nicole Weaver — Mar 4, 2012, 7:19 p.m.

Mom and I had a fun little trip to get a few things before her chemo treatments start tomorrow. We got her some warm, snuggly sweats to wear and beanies and scarves to keep her head warm. I had some gift cards, so it worked out perfectly. True to Mom and Nicki fashion, we managed to get lost in an area we have lived in for over a decade (impressive, I know). AND . . . to cheer Mom up and help her destress, I took her on a critter-petting excursion at the local pet store. They had little baby bunnies, robo hamsters, a freaky chameleon who we named "Spock," and, of course, baby lynx kittens. If anything can take the edge off, it's a mutant, six-toed, baby lynx kitten.

Mom said she had a lot of fun and it helped get her mind off things, which is what matters most. So, I am making sure to plan lots of adventures for the next few weeks, so stay tuned.

Chemotherapy Begins

By Jeff Weaver — Mar 5, 2012, 8:50 p.m.

It begins. Today was Susan's first chemo cycle. We got off to a bad start because Susan had not done her MUGA heart test because of scheduling conflicts. Consequently, the nurse would not start treatment because of the risk Adriamycin/Cytoxan (A/C) poses to Susan's heart until Susan's oncologist gave the go-ahead to proceed without the test. These drugs have very severe side effects, and heart damage is a real possibility. In fact, A/C can only be used for one cycle (four treatments) because of the risks.

To make matters worse, Susan's oncologist wasn't there, and the oncology nurse couldn't contact her by phone either. So, the nurse had to get the on-duty oncologist to sign off. However, the oncologist didn't want to take the risk or responsibility because Susan wasn't her patient. After much discussion, they finally got things straightened out. An hour later! All this didn't help Susan's stress level or the anxiety she has about taking the A/C drug.

I sat next to her and noticed how tense she was, so I thought a little humor might help take the edge off, but I was wrong. She replied in a no-nonsense manner and gave me that "enough, buddy, or you're getting it" look, so I behaved.

The oncology nurse finally brought over the red, harmless-looking bags of A/C and a bag of saline solution to wash the drug down, so to speak. Before the nurse started the treatment, she put on rubber gloves that went up to her elbows and covered Susan's arm with a towel. She told us this stuff is really toxic and they can't let it touch the skin. . . . Really! I thought, this is nuts because they are going to pump that stuff into Susan's veins.

It was all I could do to sit there and watch as the nurse inserted a big, long, fat needle into Susan's vein in the back of her hand. I hate needles, and I freak out seeing stuff like this, but it was worse for Susan because she is so small that the needle hurt her badly and the drug burned like mad. She asked the nurse repeatedly if it was supposed to hurt that much. The nurse said it was okay and that there would be some discomfort. If you ask me, it was a lot more than discomfort. And why the hell didn't the nurse use a vein in Susan's arm, like for every other patient in the place?

I have to admit that the moment the nurse shoved that needle in I realized this was really happening and, even worse, what we were facing for who knows how long. I felt bad for Susan, and I wanted to do something to help her, but at that moment there was nothing I could do.

As for Susan, well, after saying something to the nurse about the pain and burning, she didn't complain any more, but I could tell by her clenched jaw and how she squeezed her eyes shut now and again that she must be hurting. While she was getting her treatment, we talked about stuff, and for the life of me I can't remember what, even though it was just a few hours ago. And, no, it had nothing to do with being a husband who doesn't hear anything his wife says. I am guilty of that occasionally, just not this time.

When the treatment was finished, it was off to the pharmacy to get her meds. Josh was there to meet us. In the waiting area, Josh sat next to his mom, and I sat across from them. Josh looked kind of stressed and was pretty quiet, so Susan leaned over and whispered something in his ear and a big smile crossed his face. It is so typical of her to put her family first, and she wanted to make sure he was okay. I did manage to capture the moment in a photo. It was a very touching sight.

Susan will have the MUGA test tomorrow and then her CT and PET scans Wednesday and Thursday. We have our fingers and toes crossed that they show no further advancement of the cancers.

One thing Susan has to do is get a shot every day for eight days. Since she won't give herself the shots, and Josh said "hell no," and driving twenty-five miles one way to the hospital every day is out, I guess I'm going to have to do it. This could be worse than the darn chemo!

Personal Thoughts
By Jeff Weaver — Mar 7, 2012, 5:44 p.m.
Today Susan had her first scan to determine whether her cancer has spread. It's the first time she went on her own. When she got home she was subjected to the nasty side effects of her chemo treatment. I won't get into the details because it may be a little too much information and I might get in trouble.

Tomorrow she has the PET scan, and we should know the results in a few days. This is a very anxious time for all of us. I know Susan is scared to death, but she puts on a good front, even to me.

She isn't the only one who's putting on a happy face; I'm learning how to as well. I've talked to a couple friends who have gone through this, and they said to stay positive and upbeat. Makes sense to me, so that's what I will do.

None of us knows what lies ahead, and none of us are immune to the gut-wrenching times that are certainly in store for us. I am only speaking for myself, I'm a damn nervous wreck. In fact, at times it is hard for me to stay composed in her presence. I, like her, smile, make light of things, and pretend it won't be that bad, but most of all I pray to God that her cancers haven't spread and that she has the strength and willpower to fight with all she has.

And I think maybe I'm going to give myself permission to have a good cry on her shoulder. That way, maybe when she needs one she will give herself permission to cry on my shoulder. It might do both of us good.

Thanks, Everyone
By Jeff Weaver — Mar 10, 2012, 2:13 p.m.

We have just started this unwanted journey, and Susan and I are deeply appreciative of all the messages she has gotten. I am surprised by how many people have gone through something like this, because I don't think I've talked to anyone who hasn't had a close friend or family member who has had cancer.

It also gives me hope that many of them have recovered and are now leading normal lives—well, as normal as possible. That fact gives us great confidence that someday soon Susan will return to her normal routine of getting up at four thirty in the morning, driving forty-five minutes to work, stressing over whether her floors at Macy's look good enough, making sure the truckloads of new merchandise get put out and all the other things she does in her typical workday, and then spending another one to two hours in So Cal traffic to get home, where she then cares for her family and rests for twenty to thirty minutes before she goes to bed so she can get up and do it all over again. Whew, I'm tired just thinking about her "normal" day. Maybe pointing this out to her isn't such a good idea. She may delay her recovery when she remembers what normal is!

New Research
By Jeff Weaver — Mar 10, 2012, 9:37 p.m.
I just read an article written by Patrick Cox published in *The Daily Reckoning* about a new cancer drug being tested and funded by Ludwig Institute for Cancer Research in Belgium (March 9, 2012). This cancer vaccine blocks galectin-3s, proteins that identify and then "attach themselves to specific sugar molecules." Galectin-3 proteins play a big part in "strokes, heart disease, cancers, inflammation and fibrosis."

Not only do galectin-3s attach to certain sugars but they also attach to white blood cells, sometimes referred to as T cells. White blood cells defend the body against diseases and infections and send vital information to the immune system via the thymus gland, located in the middle of the chest, about the various threats.

T cells can kill cancer as long as they reach the cancerous cells. However, cancers emit galectin-3s, kind of like a "deadly fog," that hide the cancer and that then attach to the T cells, causing them to, in essence, commit suicide. Because the T cells never reach the cancer cells and gather information about the cancer, the cancers are then free to evolve and learn unabated.

So, here is the exciting part of the clinical test. When the new drug was introduced into a mix of cancer cells and T cells that had been "shut down," the result was "the T-cells were rejuvenated and began killing cancers."

This means that the new drug could be a very potent cancer killer. Very exciting stuff, I think.

Bad News
By Jeff Weaver — Mar 13, 2012, 10:10 p.m.
Susan got a call from Dr. Asuncion a few hours ago. The doctor

told her one of the scans revealed that her cancer has spread into the lymph nodes in the middle of her chest and in the abdominal region. The CT scan shows suspicious areas in her pelvic bones and in her lungs. This means Susan is at the very least stage 3 because at least one tumor has spread to the chest wall and is larger than 5 centimeters and the cancers have spread to one to three axillary lymph nodes and to the lymph nodes near the breastbone.

The doctor has ordered more scans and additional X-rays to find out for sure what the problem areas in her lungs and pelvis are. I would like to emphasize that we do not know whether this means that the cancer has spread to any of her organs.

I wish I had better news to report. We knew this wasn't going to be easy, and I hope and pray that Susan is mentally and physically prepared for what lies ahead, but this means her road just got longer and a damn sight more difficult.

Abscess and a Trip to the ER
By Nicole Weaver — Mar 15, 2012, 9:51 p.m.
Mom spent the day in the ER today because of a perineal rectal abscess. Mom had one about a year ago and was worried she might have one again. Mom is tough as nails, so typically when she has a little ache or pain, she pays it no mind. She kept saying that she felt silly being at the doctor for a little ache, but it's a good thing she listened to her body. I'm glad she went in to get it checked out, because it turns out she was right.

Mom and I got to do a lot of talking while we waited around all day for doctors and surgeons. Which for me is a treat. Mom is my best friend, so we can always find something to talk about.

It's days like today when it feels like life isn't fair and the cards are rigged in the house's favor. But it's also days like today that make me appreciate all the good things that life has to offer. Sure, no one wants to spend their day in the ER, but if you have to, who better to spend it with than the people you love the most? My friend posted a quote last night that resonated rather strongly with me today: "Life is like a roller coaster, it has its ups and downs. You can either scream or enjoy the ride." At the end of the day you have to remember that no matter how bad a hand life deals you, there is always something to be thankful for. Today I am thankful to have such amazing parents because I would not be who I am without them (okay, okay, I'm thankful for that every day).

Infection
By Jeff Weaver — Mar 15, 10:44 p.m.
I want to add a little more information about our visit to the ER today. As Nicki mentioned, about a year ago Susan had a perineal infection. These infections are painful and can cause trouble, like any infection, if not taken care of. So, when Susan told me she thought she might have another, we went straight to the ER because when we had our chemo introductory meeting we were warned that infections are very dangerous for people receiving chemotherapy.

Susan was right, and she did have another abscess. The ER doctor was a supernice man and got Susan into surgery as soon as he could so he could cut away the infected tissue. He gave her antibiotics and told us to keep a close eye on this thing because her chemo drug is very powerful and will kill lots of good cells, including her critically important white blood cells, along with the cancer cells.

I worry about Susan and antibiotics because she is allergic to several of them and has had some bad reactions in the past. We just started this and already there is trouble. God, I hope that this is a minor bump in the road.

On the way home, Susan told me that when the surgeon was done removing the infected tissue he leaned over and put his hand on her arm and said, "I know this is hard, but I really think you are going to be with us for a long time." When he said that she felt something happening in her mind, and she felt hopeful for the first time.

A Tough Weekend
By Jeff Weaver — Mar 18, 2012, 8:32 p.m.
It's Saint Patrick's Day. I am not totally up to snuff on who Saint Patrick was, other than he was kidnapped and then escaped and

became one of the most beloved saints around. But I know this other guy, Murphy, well; he didn't get a holiday, but he has a law named after him that states: "Anything that can go wrong, will go wrong."

Murphy applied his law to our household this weekend. Susan felt bad yesterday, she had no energy, and she was feeling pain where she had surgery last week. By the time she went to bed, it was getting pretty bad. Around midnight she could barely stand the pain and was in tears at times. Early this morning I took her back to the ER. Both of us were exhausted from lack of sleep.

The doctor saw lots of redness and swelling around her incision. Her white count had spiked again. The on-duty surgeon needed to go back in and clean up the newly infected area immediately because the danger was so high from this infection. The doctor couldn't wait for an operating room to open up, so that meant she couldn't put Susan under and had to use a local anesthetic instead. I must say, Susan is one tough cookie, just like Nicki said. However, she did nearly squeeze my fingers off. Bottom line is, she and my finger should survive. My finger works great now; as for her rear end, not so much.

We will have to keep a very close eye on this nasty infection. Susan's oncologist is now forced to postpone her chemo treatment until the infection is completely cleared up (about ten to fifteen days). Even though Susan's voice was weak, I heard her say, "Yay," but me, I'm a little concerned about this postponement.

This is a setback, but hopefully it will only be a small one. Now, excuse me while I go throw that Murphy fellow out on his ass!

Sometimes You're Lucky, Sometimes You're Not
By Jeff Weaver — Mar 21, 2012, 11:52 p.m.

Luck is a hard thing to put your finger on sometimes. I mean there's the luck of the draw, luck at being in the right place at the right time, and luck at winning door prizes or the lotto. But there is another kind of luck. It's the "know it when you see it" kind of luck.

This morning I was at work and got a text from Susan. She needed to go to the doctor right away. She was having a bad allergic reaction to her antibiotics. I thought, man, I can't afford to miss much more work. I know this sounds odd or like my priorities are in the wrong place, but this cancer thing is putting a real strain on our finances, and I'm really stressing over it. I worry for Susan's health, but I also worry about how I'm going to pay the rent and put food on the table. I try not to let her know about that. God knows, she has enough on her mind. She might have been able to take herself to the hospital, but what if something happened while she was driving on the freeway? So, I told my partner, David, I had to leave. I'm lucky David is such a great guy. He said, "Whatever you need. Go take care of Susan."

It's a good thing that I did take her. She was pretty wiped out from having two surgeries in a matter of three days. Her whole body was covered in thousands of bright red spots, and her back side is so tender she could barely sit. Plus, traffic was horrible, so she would have had to sit in the car for hours, but with the two of us we took the car pool lane and cut the time in half.

When we were at the check-in counter at the Mission Viejo Hospital, some guy about forty or so brought his dad in. The man was in his seventies and was having chest pains and was clearly disoriented. The lady checking him called for assistance, and two nurses rushed a wheelchair over and took him off.

We were sitting in the urgent care part of the hospital, and the place was packed. We were told the wait would be over an hour. Great, what luck, everyone in Orange County had to have an emergency today. Well, while we were waiting the guy brought his dad into the waiting room about twenty minutes later. He didn't sit next to him or even speak to him but instead sat across the room. The older man sat by himself, and it was apparent he was still very confused. He couldn't hear very well because every time a nurse came in and called out a name he would get up and ask if she was calling him. His son sat across the room, completely ignoring his father. Thirty minutes went by, and they finally called the man's name. He got up slowly and shuffled his way to the door, where the nurse escorted him to the exam rooms.

Ten minutes later the nurse came out and asked the son to come back. He got up and walked over to her, and when she told him he needed to be in with his dad, he protested. The nurse politely told him the doctor needed him back there. The guy rolled his eyes and uttered the F word. I was shocked to see his reaction.

Finally, a nurse came to get Susan and took her to an exam room. I didn't go back with her because she is very uncomfortable with me in the exam rooms when the doctors check out her . . . well, let's just say some things are better left between doctor and patient, so I went to get a drink. As I passed through the pediatrics waiting area, I saw an eight- or nine-year-old boy who was all banged up and had bloody bandages on his arms and one leg. He was sitting next to his grandfather. The grandfather tried to get up but faltered a little and nearly fell. The young boy jumped up to help his grandpa. I heard him ask if he was all right, and then he apologized for getting hurt.

I went back to the waiting room, and after a while I saw the guy come out and let the door close behind him. The door opened again, and his father came out. He was trying to find his son, who was already over at the elevator waiting for the door to open. I watched the old guy try to hurry, but he didn't make it in time and had to wait for the elevator to come back up. I was angry enough that I wanted to go give that guy a piece of my mind. Who treats their parents like that, anyway, regardless of what kind of parent they are or were? Or anyone else, for that matter.

After some time, Susan came out, and I could see she was in a lot of pain because of her two surgeries and all the poking and prodding she had to endure before and after, plus chemotherapy treatments and the reaction to the antibiotics. As she walked out she brushed her hair out of her face and looked down at her hand; it was full of her hair. Without saying anything, she just wiped it off, and I joined her. I helped Susan down the stairs to the pharmacy.

Susan and I have always been a team, and our kids are part of the team. Nicole or Josh would have gladly taken the day off if needed, and in fact they have. They've been so helpful already, and they are our best friends. I know that Susan and I will never have to suffer the indignity that guy heaped on his dad.

Sometimes we are luckier than we think.

Bacteria and Antibiotics
By Jeff Weaver — Mar 24, 2012, 11:10 a.m.

You know those things you don't pay much mind to until it affects you personally? When Susan, Nicole, and I met with her medical team, her oncologist, Dr. Asuncion, stressed to us the danger of infection. It's why she insisted that Susan not work because of her exposure to the public.

Most infections are bacterial infections, and as you know we just had a run-in with one. It really scared me because if this happened only one week after the first chemo treatment, what will the risk be after three or four of these treatments when Susan's white blood cells have been weakened or outright killed by her chemo drug? That and the fact that Susan is now allergic to at least four types of antibiotics. So, I did a little digging. Here are a few facts about bacteria:

- With five million trillion trillion of them living on Earth, they outnumber all other life-forms.
- Set end to end, they would stretch from Earth to the far edge of the universe.
- Their biomass is more than that of all plants and animals combined.
- Bacteria live in every single nook and cranny on Earth and even beyond Earth.
- Bacteria are responsible for millions of skin and soft tissue infections.
- Bacterial infections are one of America's biggest killers.
- Most bacteria are now resistant to at least one type of antibiotic.
- One of the most resistant bacteria is MRSA (methicillin-

resistant *Staphylococcus aureus*), which are among the deadliest, killing over nineteen thousand Americans in 2005.

Imagine what the statistics are in some parts of the world where sanitation is rare and medicine even rarer.

Most of us have read or heard that the overuse of antibiotics as well as their misuse to treat viral infections have resulted in bacterial resistance. That has led to a new class of superbugs that are completely immune to all antibiotics. This is becoming a very large and troublesome problem worldwide.

Even with all the warnings issued by doctors and many media outlets, I still hear far too often someone foolishly say to anyone who has a cold or the flu, "You better go to the doctor and get some antibiotics."

Just something to think about the next time you hear that from a well-intentioned but misinformed friend.

Teapots and Hair, Part One
By Jeff Weaver — Mar 25, 2012, 5:38 p.m.

This morning I crawled out of bed and went into the kitchen, filled the teapot, and turned the gas on high. I was too tired to go out and get the paper, so I just sat down and waited for the water to boil and the teapot whistle to blow.

It was a busy week, and it ended with a day we knew was coming. We have been warned about it by others, and we had watched that video provided by the doctor when we had our tour and pre-chemo meeting at the hospital.

Susan and I have spent more time in hospital emergency rooms, waiting rooms, and labs than we have at home this week. Only some of which I have chronicled. What I haven't let family and friends in on is how Susan is coping with all this. Oh, sure, I've texted Ann and Nicole a few times and let them know it might be a good idea to send a little love her way. The strain of everything she is going through is building up inside her. And the reality of her cancer diagnosis is starting to penetrate that brave front she puts up.

She had two doctor's appointments Friday, the first was at 1:00 p.m. at Sand Canyon in Irvine to have her infection checked out (so far so good) and the other was at 6:15 that evening in Anaheim (25 miles away) for her PET scan. PET scans use radioactive tracers in a special dye that are absorbed by organs and tissues. The tracers allow doctors to measure blood flow, oxygen use, and glucose metabolism (how your body uses sugar) all at the cellular level.

I came home from work to take her to the appointments. She was upset because she felt like she didn't look good. She said her hair was a mess, and she hadn't washed it since Monday because it falls out when she does wash it, and it is falling out rapidly. She had pulled it up and put one of those clippy things in the back to hold it in place. I told her she looked just fine. However, I don't think I was that convincing. There was an edge in her voice, and I knew she was getting very close to losing it.

Our plan was to go get a few things done after her first appointment and kill some time before going to Anaheim. When she got out of her first appointment it was two o'clock, and we didn't have four hours of things to keep us occupied, so we decided to go home and wait there before heading back down to her PET scan. On the way back to Diamond Bar, traffic was a nightmare due to a big wreck, so we jumped into the car pool lane and made it by this huge jam only to find that on the other side of the jam there was no way to get out of the car pool lane back into the regular lanes. As we neared our exit, I had to cross the solid double yellow lines marking the car pool lane from the regular lanes or go way up the freeway to the next exit, turn around, and drive back down to where we live.

I decided to cross over the yellow lane marker so I could get off the freeway at the exit by our house. There wasn't any traffic because of the lane closures behind us. I looked over my shoulder, checked the rearview, turned on the blinker, and eased over. We exited the freeway, and I checked my rearview mirror before stopping at the light. Crap! There was a state trooper with his red lights flashing right behind me. Apparently, when I threw Murphy out of my house last weekend, he took up residence in the car. I pulled over, and the trooper came up with his hand on his gun. I know they have to, but really, okay, not now. Anyway, I explained to the policeman what was going on with Susan and that it was either spend twenty or thirty more minutes in the car or cross the yellow line (with no one around) to get Susan home before she threw up in the car or started to bleed again. He gave me a ticket anyway and the usual lecture. I know the state is broke and they NEED their money, but, seriously, there wasn't anyone else on the highway! Needless to say, I lost it and said a few choice words about common sense and compassion—well, maybe more than a few. Susan was not happy with me, but she was less happy with the policeman. I knew I had messed up because my outburst just set her more on edge.

At five, we left for the thirty-minute drive to her second appointment at the Kaiser on Lake View, which is closer than Sand Canyon, her regular hospital. She had not eaten all day per doctor's orders and was getting hungry and shaky. For the PET scan, she was injected with the radioactive material, and then after waiting thirty minutes was given an IV with the dye. Then she had to lie motionless in the scan tube for twenty minutes. That's hard enough on its own, but Susan is still itching like mad because of her allergic reaction to her antibiotics. When she finished, I noticed how tired she looked and how much this has taken out of her.

It was another very long night for Susan. She hurts from head to toe. This is also taking a toll on me, too. I hate seeing her like this. The pain shows in her eyes, and she can barely lift her feet off the floor when she walks; she rarely holds her head up now. She spends hours curled up on the couch, and that extra spunk and sass she has always had is missing. Damn this stuff anyway.

Teapots and Hair, Part Two
By Jeff Weaver — Mar 26, 2012, 10:30 p.m.
I worked half a day, and when I got home Susan had not yet showered. She said she was exhausted because she hadn't slept much. I suggested she shower and maybe that would make her feel better. Susan and I have spent nearly twenty-six years together. I

have learned a few things along the way. Just by watching her slowly walk down the hall, her head down, and hearing how weak her voice was, but with a sharpness in her tone when she speaks, I knew she was at a low point. I have seen the tears in her eyes more than a few times this past week, but she has mostly managed to hold them in. She's pretty darn tough; however, we all remind her of that fact just in case.

While she was in the bathroom, I thought I would make myself useful and do the dishes. I waited until after she finished her shower because I have learned NEVER to turn the water on while she is in the shower. I heard her blowing her hair dry and she started swearing. Then, she heard me doing dishes by hand and the swearing turned from her hair to me. She chewed me out pretty darn good. Even though she was still inside the bathroom she got her point across loud and clear. You see, the doctor said we should always do dishes in the dishwasher because the water gets hot enough to kill any bacteria, but this time I just wanted to get them done because there weren't that many.

Next, I heard the bedroom door slam shut and thought, oops, I've done it now, so I left her alone. Then, I heard her crying. I wanted to rush in there and tell her it would be okay. But I decided she needed a good cry. And one by herself. After a while I went in and sat beside her. She was lying with her face buried in her pillow. She started crying harder and harder. I felt completely helpless, and for the life of me I couldn't think of anything to say to make her feel better. So, I just rubbed her shoulders.

Later, Nicki came over. I made some dinner, and Susan and Nicki had a nice talk. At the dinner table Susan's hair continued to fall out, and one big glob landed on her plate. We joked about her being inhabited by Rufus, our old cat that shed like no other animal on Earth. Then, Susan said it was time. She looked at Nicki and me and said we needed to cut what was left of her hair. I got out my clippers, and Nicki pulled up a chair and held her hand while I gave her a buzz cut. Susan kept repeating how hideous she was going to look. But we did manage to have a couple laughs, too. Later, Nicki and Susan sat on the couch, and Nicki pulled up some videos on how to tie a scarf on one's head. There was more laughter when they tried to tie up a silk scarf Nicki had bought Susan. Then they tried on a couple hats she had bought.

I love watching my girls when they do things together. As I cleaned the kitchen and swept up Susan's hair, I thought about everything she has been through this week and how awful some of it was and how she is starting to crack under all the pressure and stress.

Just like my teapot sitting on the flame, I knew the water would boil and the whistle would go off. And I know when Susan went off earlier, it had nothing to do with me washing the damn dishes. It was something that had to happen because the steam has been building up inside her, too. I, like usual, just provided the spark.

Good News . . . Finally
By Jeff Weaver — Mar 27, 2012, 9:47 a.m.
Yesterday Susan and I met with Dr. Asuncion, and I think we finally got some good news. According to the scans, it looks like the cancer has not spread to any other organs that we didn't already know about. However, her doctors still aren't sure about the suspicious area in her pelvic region that showed up on CT scan. And we are still waiting on the PET scan results.

So, now what? Well, Susan is going to resume her chemo treatments later this week or early next. The doctors believe they cannot afford to wait any longer because the big tumor that has grown into the chest wall is very dangerous. Susan was told that the next several weeks are going to get tough. But she was also told that after this round, the next chemo drug isn't as bad.

On another front, we are truly blessed to have so many people praying for her and rooting her on. A few people have asked me if I really believe in prayers. The answer is, I do believe in the power of prayer. Call him or her up there whatever you want, I believe we are not in this alone. I attend the Presbyterian Church of the Master in Mission Viejo, and last week after the Sunday service Nicki and I had a conversation with Pastor Jackson, and we prayed for Susan and asked God to guide us and watch over her. In fact, I have read a couple studies that dealt with people who are battling deadly diseases and whether faith has any effect on their outcomes. The answer was, yes, it does and by a healthy percentage. One reputable study found that 65 percent of the participants in the group who believed in the power of prayer had better results than those in the group who did not believe in the power of prayer.

All I know for sure is it helps me cope with this, and I know it sure as heck doesn't hurt.

Rain
By Jeff Weaver — Apr 1, 2012, 1:31 p.m.
It rained last night in So Cal . . . again . . . and I wasn't too happy about it. Thinking about that strikes me as funny; after all, I did grow up in Oregon, where it rained all the time. You could count on 26 to 30 inches of rain in Douglas County and on the South Umpqua River flooding every other year. In Brookings, where Susan grew up, it rains 120-plus inches every year.

For some reason the rain this morning reminded me of when we moved to Las Vegas in January of 1997 to open a new financial planning office. It was the start of a journey that I had willingly decided to take (after convincing Susan that I knew what I was doing). I was taking a big risk moving so far away from family and friends and starting over again.

We had a lot of help moving. My good friend, Mike Carter, came over and brought a friend whose job was loading moving trucks. Mike, Susan, and I spent all day packing boxes from the house to the truck. The kids pitched in, too. Early the next morning we hit the road and began our new adventure. My dad helped us by driving one of the cars, and Susan, the other, while I drove the U-Haul loaded down with everything we owned.

It took us two days to get to Las Vegas and most of one day to unload the truck and get everything into the new house. We were exhausted. I remember sitting at the table that evening, tired and sore, eating Big Macs and fries. Susan and my dad gave me a bunch of guff about driving too fast on the 15 Freeway that morning and losing them in all the downtown Vegas traffic. I still contend that Susan, driving her Mustang GT, and my dad, driving my Thunderbird SC, should have been able to keep up with a big, clunky, loaded-down 26-foot U-Haul. But then, they didn't know the area or how to drive in city traffic. As we sat at the table, we laughed and enjoyed those Big Macs. We were family after all.

I tell you this because that first morning in our new house when I got up, I saw Dad standing alone at the window looking out at the desert sky. It was raining. And it must have made him homesick. Maybe all he could think of were his cows back home on the farm. He was worried about having someone else taking care of them, and he missed Mom. Dad is a farm boy, and a little uncomfortable in the city. I tried to tell him it would be okay on the farm. But it didn't work, so later I took him down to the airport and got him on an early stand-by flight home. All Dad wanted was to be home with his wife and where he was in control and felt comfortable and safe.

✿

Anyway, after I put on the coffee, I walked out to get the Sunday paper. I stopped and looked up at the sky. The clouds were thick and dark. The rain had soaked my paper even though it was wrapped in a protective orange plastic bag. I took a deep breath and stood in the rain, and suddenly I felt homesick. Maybe at that moment I needed my dad to tell me everything was going to be okay and that I was doing the right things for Susan. I just stood there looking up at the dark clouds hanging over my house, and the raindrops were hitting my face. I felt them run down my cheeks, where they mingled with tears as I thought about this new journey my family has just started. A journey of unknown length and destination.

And for the first time in a very long time I felt lost and unsure.

Tuesday Susan starts her chemo treatments again. I remembered what the doctor told us this week when she reminded us this is going to be a tough slog and Susan was going to get really sick but that it would get easier later on.

As I turned to walk back into the house, I glanced at the horizon through the rain. The clouds had parted ever so slightly, and I saw a small ray of light beaming down. It reminded me that with all the prayers from friends and family we will get through this . . . and God will help us find our way.

But first we must walk through a little rain.

The Worst Possible News
By Jeff Weaver — Apr 2, 2012, 10:27 p.m.
Today Susan had an appointment with her oncologist, Dr. Asuncion. We both thought this was for her pre-chemo bloodwork and to check on the infection. I didn't go with her because I was sure this was routine.

We were wrong. The news Susan got was devastating. Dr. Asuncion told her that both her cancers have spread to the bones in her pelvic area and in her chest. She was told she is now stage 4.

I took some time to think this through and try to sort things out. Later, I went outside and called Dr. Asuncion because I needed to hear from her what this really meant for Susan. She said she was going to change the strategy. Instead of chemo every two weeks, Susan was going to go every three weeks. They are changing the drugs that they will use after Susan finishes the round of A/C. I asked Dr. Asuncion why slow down now? Why not try to kick this thing's butt? She said it was now a quality-of-life issue rather than a kill-the-cancer issue.

Dr. Asuncion said the only choice she had now is to try to control the cancer rather than kill it because they can't, so she has to treat it as a chronic disease. Then, I asked her to tell me the truth about what all this means. She told me that because Susan's cancers are incurable, Susan has maybe three to five years to live, but that it is the doctor's hope to make her as comfortable as possible and do everything she can to extend Susan's life for as long as possible.

It was so hard to tell Susan what I had just heard. The look on her face told me she was terrified. There was total silence in the room.

We stood there all alone, each with our own thoughts, holding each other. I felt her heart pounding. We didn't say anything because I don't think either of us knew what to say.

I had to call Susan's folks because she said she couldn't. I think it was even harder to tell Ann and Martin this awful news. They have already lost their only son in an auto accident several years ago. Now I tell them they may lose their only daughter. I wish we could have told them in person. I called my dad after that and let him know. He was pretty shook up as well. He and Susan have a great relationship. Next, I called Nicki, and that didn't go well. Both Susan and I talked to Josh, and he was shaken. I can't imagine what is going through their minds.

I am mentally exhausted. I am afraid, afraid of what is next and what other bad things may yet come our way. Why the hell is this happening to us?

I know a lot of people are praying for Susan, and I think she needs the prayers now more than ever. One thing is for sure, though. Along with being scared, I'm mad, so I'm rolling up my sleeves and I'm going to work to find every way possible to help Susan fight her cancer.

Calling All Angels
By Jeff Weaver — Apr 5, 2012, 12:38 p.m.
For the past couple days Susan and I have been struggling with the reality of this whole thing. Needless to say, it has been a very emotional and confusing time. There are so many questions we don't have answers to, and every day still more questions pop up. We feel like we have somehow lost control. I know I feel totally helpless. But I have to do something. I don't care what it takes, I'll do my best to find something that will help her. And I hope and pray Susan is up for the tough fight she has in front of her.

Last night Susan said something that I think a few of us are thinking. She said, "This just isn't fair." Then she asked me, "What have I done to deserve this? I've never smoked or drank or done drugs. I've tried to take care of myself."

It's a fair question and one that has no good answer. At least not one I can come up with. And believe me, I have been asking that same question. The only thing I can think of is that this is not about fairness. If it was, then she would not have cancer. But that doesn't keep us from wondering why.

And, for the first time, we had a conversation about her mortality. I have often thought about mine because I've had many brushes with death over the years and I am getting to the age when a lot of us start pondering our mortality. I'm sure we will have many talks about the subject as we go forward.

It struck me this morning on my way to work that this weekend is Easter Sunday and if ever there was a time to think about such things and search for answers, this Sunday is a good time to start.

As I mentioned, we are not going to take this sitting down. We will not give in to this disease. We are going to start with diet because I've come across many studies and articles about cancer and food. I am going to start researching what she should be eating and what she should not. Research is something I like doing, so I will dive in head first.

Another thing we will do is make sure we stay focused on the important things in life, like family and friends. This Sunday we will be focusing on our faith and spiritual well-being.

And after church, Josh is taking me to the Angels opening weekend game versus the Kansas City Royals. For those who have never attended an Angels game, they always start by playing "Calling All Angels."

Rather appropriate, I'd say!

Kindness
By Jeff Weaver — Apr 6, 2012, 10:26 p.m.
We know there will be good days and bad days as Susan travels the road she is now on. We don't know what lies around the next corner, but we know what's at the end of her journey. It is the same end we all have eventually. And everyone's road will have a few bumps, and their journey will have a surprise or two along the way. Some of

those surprises will be wondrous and humbling.

Today is a really bad day for Susan. The drug that runs through her is kicking her rear end pretty good. But I don't want to talk about that now. I want to talk about yesterday. It may not have been the best day of her life, but it ranks right up there.

Susan and I and the kids, too, have been under enormous stress for a while, and not all of it is due to Susan's disease. After we got the last bit of terrible news, I've been worried about her and kind of waiting for her to lose it emotionally. I have spent as much time in prayer as in anything else I do. I pray that she won't hurt and be too sick, or sometimes I just pray for something good to happen, anything at all.

Yesterday, after I got home from work, I was sitting in my chair feeling a little down. Susan was not feeling very good and was lying on the couch, so I picked up the newspaper and tried to read it. Josh came home from work and brought the mail in with him. He had an unmarked envelope along with several cards. He handed everything to Susan. In the mail there was a letter from her mom. Susan opened the letter from Ann, and out of the corner of my eye I saw her holding a check, and she was crying. Not full-on crying, but I thought it was time for it, so I let her be.

Then, she started opening the cards. They were from her Macy's family. With each card she read, there were tears, and then she opened the unmarked envelope. She broke down completely. I asked her what was wrong, and she just stared at the envelope crying. After a few minutes she handed it to me. I was shocked at what I saw. It was full of money that her friends from work had given her.

Once in a great while we witness extraordinary acts of kindness. Yesterday Susan and I saw that kindness first hand. We cannot possibly thank her mom and her Macy's family enough. It was truly moving and very humbling. And it turned out to be a wondrous day.

Susan said the least she can do is bake some cookies for her friends at Macy's, or, if she is too sick, I will.

Heroes, Part One
By Jeff Weaver — Apr 10, 2012, 9:40 a.m.

Yesterday I needed a break, and as I often do when I have free time, I write. Mostly, I just jot down ideas or work on projects I have already started. One of my projects is a story about heroes titled "Gemstones and Heroes." I had my notebook out and was going over some hand-written notes, adding thoughts here and there. Susan was on the couch resting when she got a call on her cell phone. I heard her answer in a voice that made me look up.

She sounded surprised and, I must say, really excited. I thought, wow, who could that be? She had a big smile on her face and she was animated. Whoever it was asked Susan how she was feeling. She said she was doing good and had been a "little tired" for a day or two. They talked and laughed. It was great.

To put the record straight, though, she was not a "little tired"; she was wiped out and sick as heck. For a good part of the last two days, Susan has been lying on the couch wrapped in an electric blanket with her eyes closed, shivering and shaking from the effects of the chemo treatments. I can't put into words how hard it is to see her like this.

When she got off the phone, I asked her who that was, and she said Maria Dennehy, her store manager. I commented on how thoughtful it was that her boss called, because I know how many hours store managers put in each day and how many problems they deal with day in and day out. Then Susan and I talked again about how her Macy's family has responded to all this and their generosity and how much she misses them.

I looked down at my notebook. At the top of the page was something I had written for a poetry class. It was only three short lines that had to define something—I had chosen heroism—but we had to use poetic conventions.

"Heroism is a sacrifice / whose action / of selflessness supersedes self." Then I thought about everything Susan's friends had done for her. I want to remind everyone that retail isn't the highest-paying gig out there; far from it. And it struck me that her friends at Macy's had made such a sacrifice, and in my book, that makes them heroes.

I heard the timer on the oven ding. We got up, and Susan went over to the oven and pulled out dinner. We sat down and enjoyed a meal prepared for us a few days ago by one of Susan's closest friends and coworker, Francesca Capella. She wanted us to have something we could freeze and heat up when time was short or we didn't feel like cooking. It was delicious!

Heroes, Part Two
By Jeff Weaver — Apr 11, 2012, 5:41 p.m.

So, how do we define a hero anyway? Well, I looked up the word and found this: "A hero is someone who helps without anything expected in return. Their gesture may be big or small, profound or not." Sounds like Ann and Marty, and the Macy's crew, as well as those who leave Susan notes on her website and those who pray for her.

Then there is this definition in another dictionary: "A person distinguished by exceptional courage and nobility and strength." It is this hero I want to talk about today. But first I need to provide some background.

I'm not that good at a lot of things, but one thing I am good at is seeing people for who they really are and being able to find the good in nearly everyone I meet (Susan says this is also a fault of mine once in a while). And I know a good thing when I see it.

Anyone believe in love at first sight? Well, I do, and I knew it when I first set eyes on Susan. It was in 1985, and she was in a small gym in Brookings, Oregon. I was working out when I first saw her, and I had to stop doing whatever it was I was doing. I stood there like a dumbstruck kid and just stared at her. She turned her head toward me and gave me this look. Her eyes were so blue, and she was the most beautiful girl I had ever seen. I have been madly in love with her from that moment. And our love affair with each other continues to this day. Sure, there have been a few rocky times, but we never doubted each other's love.

Over the years I've learned what kind of person she really is.

Temperamental, for sure, but also fair. She is kind and generous, she truly cares for people, she has a work ethic like few others, she is smart and witty, she is honest to a fault, and she is a down-to-earth girl, not a "fancy" girl, if you know what I mean. She's also loyal, a great mom, and she has been all any man could ask for in a lifelong partner.

Lately, I have seen another side of her. I have watched as she has put the needs of others before her own even as she fights for her life. I've seen her comfort others. Even after she got the worst news a person could get, I saw a level of compassion in her I didn't know was there.

Last week a good friend, Mike Gray, called me. Now, Mike and his wife, Melissa, are religious people, and a few months ago they were in a terrible car wreck and Melissa was hurt badly. Anyway, Mike told me that they were praying for Susan, and he asked me how she was doing. Susan was standing next to me, so I said, why not ask her? and handed the phone to Susan. They had a long talk about her cancer, Melissa, and God. When they finished, Susan handed the phone back to me. Mike was struggling for words. He said he had called to cheer her up, and what had happened was she cheered him up instead. He said he couldn't believe how upbeat and caring someone could be after the news she got.

Then, last Friday I saw something that is hard to talk about, or even write about, but I'll try. We have all seen the "brave" front folks put on at times. Susan is getting darn good at it. For one thing, she has to endure me giving her shots right before bed. Let me tell you, she deserves a medal just for that. Susan has been really sick and she is in a lot of pain, but she doesn't complain about it. Oh sure, she will say something but more in a matter-of-fact way. After all our years together, I've learned to read her facial expressions. So, I know when she feels bad and I bet I could tell you just how bad, too. It was bedtime, so that meant shot time. I got the needle out of the fridge and was walking across the living room to where she was sitting on the couch all slumped down. She looked exhausted and her jaw was kind of clenched because of the pain she was in.

But still, she managed a smile when she saw me because she knows how much I hate giving her those darn shots. And sure enough, this one didn't go well. I hit a nerve or something because she cried out and jumped. Freaked me out! She patted me on the leg and said, "I'm sorry."

We got up and walked down the hall. Susan looked like she was going to collapse, so I walked behind her. She went into the bathroom, turned on the water, and stood bent over the sink splashing her face with the warm water, over and over. It kills me that she hurts so much and that I can't help her. I left her alone so she could finish her nightly routine and went to bed.

When Susan came into the bedroom, she was in her PJs and had taken off her stocking cap. The light was out in our room, but the light in Josh's room across the hall was on. When she turned to shut the door, I could see her profile. It was like I was looking at an old black-and-white photograph. Parts of her face were dark and parts were highlighted by the dim, soft light coming from Josh's room. Her head looked tiny without hair. She looked delicate and beautiful. I couldn't take my eyes off her. Then she turned to me and in the semidarkness I again saw how tired she was and how much pain she was in. I could see the dark circles under her eyes, and I noticed she was losing weight. She sat down on the bed, took a deep breath, and exhaled slowly. She labored to lift her legs up onto the bed and pull the covers over her. Her head sank into the pillow. She didn't say a word. I lay there looking at her, and I saw tears run down her cheek. My heart was breaking. With her eyes closed she reached over and took my hand and held it for the longest time.

Let me ask you, doesn't that sound like a person distinguished by exceptional courage and nobility and strength? She is my hero, that much is for sure.

An Ounce of Prevention
By Jeff Weaver — Apr 14, 2012, 11:17 a.m.
I am always looking for new information about cancer, and I came across a piece by Deepak Chopra titled "Is Cancer Ready for a Turn

Around?" (SFGate, April 8, 2012). It was very insightful.

The article states that the Centers for Disease Control and Prevention reported "that two-thirds of cancers may be preventable." The report found that the main causes of these preventable cancers are smoking and obesity along with lack of exercise. These are lifestyle choices we have control over.

Here are a few other quotes from the piece.

"The MD Anderson Cancer Center in Houston went so far as to consider 90–95% of cancers preventable."

"Serious attention is now going to 'belly fat,' which triggers hormones like insulin and estrogen as well as inflammatory compounds throughout the body." These are all significant causes of cancer.

The article also cited three new studies that found aspirin is still one of the best anti-inflammatories on the market. That is important because chronic inflammation is a serious danger to human health because it damages cells at the DNA level by releasing inflammation-induced chemicals into the body that are directly related to "cancerous tumors."

So, what can we do to reduce chronic inflammation? Turns out, quite a lot, and it doesn't cost a thing, other than a little time and willpower. Lifestyle choices are the key. Exercise daily because that helps get rid of the killer belly fat and helps overall weight reduction, increases energy levels, and improves cardiovascular health, which helps get more oxygen and nutrients to the cells. Eat right by increasing the amount of whole grains, vegetables, dark greens, and fruit in our diet and reduce red meat and sugar consumption. Also reduce stress and take a few minutes every day to meditate.

I know what many will say: "Well, I know so-and-so who drank, smoked, and ate beef every day and he/she lived to be ninety-five." I know people just like that myself; my family is full of them. However, to put this into context, the next generation will be the first generation ever to have shorter lifespans than their parents. So, it seems to me if we continue to ignore the benefits of making positive lifestyle changes, it's like playing Russian roulette with two live rounds in a six-shot revolver.

There is no escaping that making wholesale lifestyle changes is radical for most of us, but we also cannot escape the fact that it is good for us, it can and will extend our lives, and we will have more disease-free and healthy years. With all the new research being done on lifestyle, it is becoming plainly evident the reasons for practicing prevention grow more powerful every day.

Susan and I are implementing many of the aforementioned lifestyle changes. Exercising, taking time to meditate, eating right, and, of course . . . taking an aspirin a day, hoping it keeps cancer away.

Talkin' Food
By Jeff Weaver — Apr 17, 2012, 11:18 p.m.

There has been a change. Not in a bad way; this change is positive. It has nothing to do with the diagnosis, but I think it will change the prognosis.

In the last entry I shared some general information about the effects of holistic treatments and how diet plays such a big part in people's health. I decided to call an old friend and another of my life mentors, John Liviakis. Right before I was diagnosed with cancer, I went to work for John up in Mill Valley. He owned the premier corporate communications firm in the world. John is the most driven man I have ever met. He is also an expert on holistic diets and the health benefits of whole foods. I told John all about Susan and asked him for help. He told me about new food-based supplements that are being tested that show real promise, and he gave me direction on plant-based diets.

Then I did more reading and research. It appears that diet may be the single biggest reason why some folks survive cancer and other diseases, and some don't.

So, this weekend Susan and I made the commitment to do whatever it takes, no matter how difficult it is, and that includes changing our diet.

This isn't like some weight-loss diet where you can cheat once in a while. This is a matter of life and death, to put it bluntly. That raises the stakes some. It's also a matter of responsibility because Susan and I feel a responsibility to Josh and Nicole, Ann and Marty, and to everyone who has prayed for her and been so generous with their time and money. She told me, "If they can do everything they have done, the least I can do for them is to fight as hard as I can."

The first thing I did was put together which foods go on our do-not-eat list, or the list of "stuff that got us here in the first place." It's a big list! Then I made a list of good things to eat. (You can find them later in the Foods, Spices, and Herbs section.) I thought, heck, I like this stuff. Susan and I sat down to go over the changes. This is kind of how it went:

I said, "Hey, this ain't gonna be so bad. Lots of fresh fruit and veggies. Look, it says right here papaya is a superfood."

"Really," she said. "I don't like papaya. Tastes like crap."

"Crap? No, honey, this stuff is really good for you . . . you'll see. I bet I can fix it where you'll love it. Maybe with some mango and pineapple, with a little ginger. . . . I'll make a chutney. . . . I'll chiffonade some fresh mint and basil and use that for a garnish . . . you'll see."

"Don't like papaya. Tastes like crap. What else ya got?"

I looked across the table and she was sitting there with the warm afternoon sun reflecting off her cute, bald head. "Well, let's see, we can cook up a mess of cruciferous vegetables, like brussels sprouts and broccoli, oh . . . oh . . . and dark leafy greens like kale and collard greens or maybe some turnips and radishes and cabbage. . . ."

"Are you crazy? When have you ever seen me eat that stuff? Tastes like crap. . . . Come on, what else?"

"Hmm," I said. "Well, how about some tasty, tender carotenoids? I could julienne some red and yellow and orange peppers, throw in a little onion, and toss them with some fresh lemon juice."

"What are you tryin' to do, give me heartburn or something? You know I can't eat peppers. Besides, anything with lemon or lime tastes like crap since I started chemo. Too acidic."

"You know, you better put that wool hat back on your shiny dome or it's gonna get sunburned. Remember, you burn real easy now." And I quickly looked back down at all the research papers spread out in front of me. "Damn, let's see . . . oh . . . oh . . . I could take leafy greens, broccoli sprouts, a few alfalfa sprouts, and spinach and Swiss chard and mix 'em with sunflower greens . . . and put them in that new juicer David gave us, or I could make you some wheatgrass juice or maybe a tall, cold glass of barley grass juice," I said proudly and looked up at her.

"Geeezzz, Jeff, do you think I'm a cow or something? How about finding something I can eat, for Pete's sake!"

"Don't have to be so snippy with me," I said. "Okay, ever eat seaweed? They got lots of different ones. There's the nori and kombu, wakame or that dulse seaweed . . . that's yummy, I hear, especially drizzled with some flaxseed oil and topped with a few sardines or mackerel."

"Okay, smart guy, even *you* think that stuff tastes like crap. Isn't there anything good?"

"But, baby [I still call her baby], I know I can make all this stuff taste like . . . like . . . chicken. You know me, give me some fresh ingredients and I'll come up with something good."

"Yeah, like those big, thick juicy steaks you used to grill and slather with butter and blue cheese sauce. Now that was good," she said, with that mischievous smile of hers plastered all over her face.

"Funny," I said, and picked up my sunglasses and put them on. "Sorry, the sun is glaring off your shiny bald head, dear."

"What else ya got?"

"Hmm, maybe I better do a little more research. Says here that you have to be even stricter with your diet while you're on chemo. . . . I'll have ta' get back to you on this."

Of course, that's only how I remember the conversation, and thank God Nicki showed up and saved my bacon—oh, I forgot . . . we can't have bacon. It's got sodium phosphates, sodium erythorbate, and that evil sodium nitrite in it, not to mention tons of regular salt and sugar.

All joking aside, this diet thing is huge, and there will be wholesale changes at our house.

Determination
By Nicole Weaver — Apr 19, 2012, 7:32 p.m.

I am terrible at math and accidentally signed myself up for a five-unit algebra class, thinking it was *pre* algebra. I immediately considered dropping the class; however, the professor's lecture the first night really caught my attention. First, he said we would have homework, but he didn't collect it. In my head I'm thinking I just lucked into the best math class ever. Then, he said something that made me stop and think, actually *think*!

"Why are you taking this class?"

Simple enough, right? *I'm taking this class so I can graduate from college.* Wrong.

My professor kept asking things like, "Well, why do you want to graduate college? Why do you want a good-paying job? Why? Why? Why? . . . " Until finally he said, "Listen, the secret to discipline is remembering what you REALLY want." Hence, the reason he does not collect homework. He believes that if you truly want something, you will do it.

I read the journal entry my dad wrote about the new diet and the choices we make in life, and I thought, hmm, Professor Barry is onto something here. For the first time in my life I am actually doing my homework on time and willingly because every time I don't feel like doing it, I think about why I am REALLY taking this class. I don't know how relevant this is to this whole journey, but it is such a simple idea, and it has had a big impact on my thinking, so I wanted to share it. And I know my mom really wants to stick around.

Changing Doctors
By Jeff Weaver — Apr 20, 2012, 8:44 p.m.

Susan met with Dr. Asuncion today, and she told us Susan would be getting a new oncologist. Dr. Asuncion is transferring up to LA to be closer to where she lives. She has recommended Dr. Rupali, a young doctor who trained at UCLA.

Susan is upset by this development. Not because of the new doctor, but because she is losing Dr. Asuncion. I haven't written much about Dr. Asuncion, but we like her a lot and trust her more. Susan has a real connection with her, and I think that it goes both ways.

It will be a couple months before Dr. Asuncion leaves. We didn't really need this now.

But this is another example of how little control you have when you fight a disease like cancer. We will deal with it and do the best we can and most of all pray that Dr. Rupali is as good as Dr. Asuncion.

Praying for Better Days
By Jeff Weaver — Apr 21, 2012, 11:42 a.m.
I just got in from a walk. I walk for the exercise. But walking also helps clear my mind and it helps me think. Most of the time I take our black, white, and copper Aussie, Mick, with me. He likes walking more than I do, and even though he is eight years old, he still acts like a puppy. I like talking to Mick on our walks. I know he hears me, too, because he always looks back over his shoulder when I speak to him. Lately, though, I have been talking more with God, and Mick seems to be okay with that.

I needed the walk more than ever this morning because I have so much on my mind these days, and most of it is troubling. My job, which is commission only, has been tough for the past three months. I work fifty or more hours a week in a dying industry, so I go for long stretches with no income. I am working out the details of our new diet in which every ingredient has to have some cancer-fighting property and am trying to make everything taste good. I do hours of research on new treatments and supplements that might help Susan. She is the last thing I see when I finally go to bed. When she takes off her hat and I see her with no hair, I am conflicted because she is beautiful but also seeing her like that forces the reality of this on me.

I can't sleep because I worry and, frankly, because I am afraid.

And to top it off, this week I was told by my doctor that I have degenerative arthritis in most of my joints, and that the joints in my toes, fingers, back, and knees are beyond help, and that the sharp stabbing pain in my sinus cavity where I had bone removed in two surgeries is chronic, and that there is absolutely nothing they can do about it. . . . Well, there was the "go home and take two aspirin" thing . . . whoopee! Like I haven't already tried that one.

As I headed out the door this morning, I looked up at the sky, and the fog was thick, and I could still feel the heat from yesterday hanging in the air. I thought, oh, great, it is going to be nearly a hundred degrees today and humid.

So, off Mick and I went. He was thrilled. As long as he gets fed, petted, and walked, he's a happy boy. He especially likes it when he gets to go out early when the air is clean and fresh and the night scents are still lingering on the morning breeze. Mick is full of energy and doesn't have a worry in the world. He walks off leash because he is so well trained, and there are times when I hardly know he's with me. This morning was like that.

As we headed up the steep hill at the start of our walk, the joints in my toes felt like someone was stabbing me with an ice pick, and a pain was shooting down my lower back all the way to my knee because of an injury I suffered in the Army that damaged my lower spine. Each step was pure agony. I thought, the heck with this, I'm turning back. I stopped and slumped my shoulders. I was feeling sorry for myself. Mick heard me, or rather didn't hear me walking, so he stopped and looked back at me (he likes to lead the way). The smile he had turned into something like a worried look. He tilted his head to the right, then he ran back to me and touched my finger with his nose, then he circled around me and ran out in front of me and begged me to continue.

I looked up into the heavens and I asked, "God, why is all this happening to me?"

Then God's voice came to me. He said, "Why not? Are you special? Would you rather be in Susan's shoes?"

Without even thinking, I said, "Yes, please make her well and give it to me. I'll gladly trade places. I know I am good at fighting things like that. Remember, I've done it before and beat it."

"That's not how this works," he said. "I don't pick and choose who gets sick or who lives and dies. I just offer peace in this life and life after death."

"Peace!" I said. "What about a little peace now? Haven't you heard any of my prayers?"

"Sure I have . . . all of them, and I also remember you asking me why you were put on this earth. How many times now, hundreds? I've heard you tell Susan and many others that you knew there was a reason why you are here and that is why you have survived all those encounters with death. You said you had a purpose, a destiny."

"Well, maybe so, but you know I was thinking something big, something that would change people's lives."

"Hmm," God said in a soft, thoughtful voice.

"I want to ask something of you," I said. "Let's see if I can put it in words, let me try to make it clear. . . . I just want Susan to see better days. We don't need much money or fancy things. We would like to be in a place where life is simple and . . . fair." I looked back down at Mick. He was sitting, his tongue out and his head still tilted. He was listening to me intently. I looked back up. "Look, God, all I want now is for Susan to get well. And that she doesn't suffer—"

"Do you believe in me?" he interrupted.

"Sure I do, you know that."

"No, I mean really believe."

"Well, yeah, I think I do. Although, to be honest, I do have doubts at times, but then don't we all?"

"Most do, but not those who are all in. You asked for peace, for better days. You asked why you're here. Maybe you should finish your walk, take inventory of what you *do* have, look around . . . pay attention to what you see, listen to what others are saying, and then give it all a think. Remember, I am always here if you need to talk."

"Okay, I will. And thanks for the time," I said, not wanting to push my luck.

"No problem. Oh, by the way, I hear a lot of prayers coming from a lot of people. Seems that Susan has many friends. She's lucky, you know."

Mick came over and touched my finger again with his wet nose. He whirled and took off, stopped and looked back over his shoulder. "Well, you coming or are you gonna quit?"

Fighting Addiction
By Jeff Weaver — Apr 23, 2012, 2:01 p.m.

We're addicted, much like a smoker or an alcoholic or drug addict. But it's not cigarettes or whiskey or some sinister drug. It's chocolate chip cookies, it's cheeseburgers and french fries, and it's pizza that we are hooked on.

Susan and I are finding out this addiction is real, whether it be mental or, as I suspect, physical. We find ourselves craving these foods. Susan and I went on the new diet where we are eliminating animal proteins and dairy and sugar and all fried foods. I have done hours of research trying to find any study that tells us that meat and dairy will improve our general health or, more to the point, will help fight and reverse her cancer. Sadly, I haven't found a single study by a nonpartisan group that concludes that a glass of milk or a beef steak or grilled chicken breast will extend our lives or fight cancer, despite the millions of dollars spent by the lobby groups of those industries. However, I have found dozens of studies that show plant-based diets that are high in antioxidants and other proven cancer-fighting elements can prevent and, in some cases, reverse cancer.

On the advice from my business partner, David, Susan and I watched the video *Forks Over Knives*. It was eye-opening and gave us a lot of information on how to best eat for health. One thing I want to be careful about is becoming an annoying advocate of one diet over another. I will try not to sound like I am preaching at folks. Diet, like religion, is a personal choice.

The problem for Susan is this: she has to make a change. She simply cannot eat the way she did. Science is clear that cancer needs certain things to survive; chief among them is sugar, red meat, and hydrogenated oils. Without going into the studies on that now, we believe that we must cut them from our diet.

Susan must "starve" the cancer to death and reduce the artificially caused cellular inflammation or it will end up killing her.

Harsh statement? Sure it is, but it is also a true statement. And that brings me back to our addiction. We love chocolate chip cookies, cheeseburgers, and pizza. And, like any addict, we get weak and we think about what we cannot have more than what we can. For example, we went grocery shopping Saturday with our list. It was all stuff that is on the strict new plan, lots of leafy greens, fruits, veggies, beans, whole grains, and other like items. On the way we passed an In-N-Out Burger joint. Those of you in California know how good their burgers are . . . they're legendary! Susan said, oh, stop, please, I want one. My response: sorry, dear, no can do. Next we were at a stoplight and to the right was a Round Table Pizza place. We could smell the pepperoni . . . oh, please, can we stop here? No, dear.

As we drove to Sprouts, it was one place after an another: BBQ joints, burger chains, taco stands, pizza places, and bakeries . . . all calling us, speaking to our addictions . . . assuring us that just one more time won't hurt.

The point is, this is going to be HARD. In part, because we are *forced* to radically change our diets (if we want to give Susan the best shot at living) rather than *wanting* to do it.

On the way home from the market, we passed the Round Table again. People were coming and going—families, couples, Little League baseball teams—and they all looked like they were having a good time. Susan said, "Damn it, I want pizza."

When we got home we carried our sacks of veggies and fruits and whole-grain foods into the house. Susan sat down while I went to make her dinner. I had a little surprise in store for her.

Twenty-five minutes later, I hollered, "Dinner's ready, and it looks GOOD, baby."

She came in, and sitting on the table was my version of pizza—a vegetarian pizza on a whole-grain crust and no cheese.

"Wow, this looks good, honey, and it smells great."

"Thanks, baby. Hope you like it."

It was awesome, and every ingredient had some cancer-fighting component to it. Susan loved it and so did I. After dinner she sat back on the couch, and I heard, "I want a chocolate chip cookie."

"Junkie!" I said.

Spraying to All Fields
By Jeff Weaver — Apr 25, 2012, 4:15 p.m.
Yesterday Susan had her third chemo treatment and that means she has one more round with this drug. In the middle of May, she will be evaluated by her oncologist, and at that time we will find out what the next cycle of treatments will be and whether the current drugs have had any effect on her tumors. So far, there has been no change in her markers.

I went with her to keep her company. After we waited in the lobby for ten minutes, the nurse came out to get us. Susan had a new nurse, Diane, who was supernice and who made Susan feel as comfortable as possible before she put in the IV and started the two-hour drip of A/C.

I noticed a new sign on the nurse's station wall; it was a reprint from a piece in *US News & World Report* that ranked hospitals in the different specialties. Sand Canyon Kaiser is ranked way up there in the cancer category. It is comforting to know Susan has some of the best care available.

The diet is coming along, but we must plan meals ahead. For example, yesterday after Susan's chemo treatment we needed to get something to eat. We are discovering that we can't eat at most places. She can't eat anything raw while she is on chemo, so no salads or fresh fruits. Most places put too much salt and sugar in their food (we are serious about this sugar thing). Finding places on the fly does not work! So, from now on we will do a little research on restaurants in an area before we go. But, on the other hand, we are finding that the meals we make at home for the most part are very good. And we don't really miss the dairy and meat . . . yet.
Spirits Flying High

And Now We Fight

By Jeff Weaver — Apr 26, 2012, 11:31 p.m.

One of the most import things you can do when you are in a battle with advanced cancer is to make sure you stay positive and keep your spirits up. But this is a lot harder to do than you might think. I know when I was fighting cancer it was a constant battle to stay positive, and I think it is for Susan, too.

It is hard to properly describe to someone how sick cancer treatments make you and how much pain you are in. And I am sure when I try to write about it here, there are many who think I'm being a bit melodramatic. But that's not the case. Cancer sucks the life out of you, literally and figuratively. The treatments are awful.

Lately, Susan has been hit by cancer's one-two punch: the disease is trying to take away her will, her mental strength, and her life, while the treatments are making her hurt all over and making her feel extremely sick twenty-four hours a day . . . day after day.

But sometimes relief comes from unexpected places. Yesterday I got an email from Drew Hilliard. I don't know Drew nor have I ever heard of him. But his email was extraordinary, and it was just what the doctor ordered.

So, who is Drew? Well, turns out he is a young Navy lieutenant from Louisville, Kentucky. Drew heard about Susan's fight with cancer from my niece, Sandra, and her husband, Nate Dishman. Drew is also in a fight for his life with a rare form of cancer, sarcoma, I believe. He knows what it's like and how hard it is. So, he took time to send Susan a photo of himself holding a big sign. It reads: "Thinking of and praying for you, Susan! Lieutenant Drew Hilliard."

I was very moved by this, and I called Susan into my writing room and showed her the photo. She was speechless. I saw her tear up. Finally, she asked me who he was. I told her and we both just looked at the picture for a while. She asked me why someone would do this. The best answer I had was that everyone who has cancer is in a very special club, like it or not, and we all root openly for each other.

Then today I got another email, this time from my niece, Sandra Dishman. She sent along a photo of her husband and two of his

Navy fighter pilot buddies. They are standing in front of a fighter jet, and they too are holding a sign. It said, "Susan, we are proud to serve and fight for you! God bless you and your family. Dirty - T Bone - Dolph."

I showed it to Susan and she was very moved by this. I wrote Drew and Sandra emails, thanking them for their inspirational gestures.

So, it looks like Susan now has the U.S. Navy on her team. These men are the real deal and real warriors, who have put their lives on the line for our country.

Susan too is a warrior who is in a fight for her life. These pictures have lifted her sprits, and both she and I pledge to fight her cancer any way we can and with all the resolve we can muster.

It Ain't Over
By Jeff Weaver — Apr 27, 2012, 10:55 a.m.

We are at the very beginning of this journey, and all of us want this to be over. We know Susan's doctors do not have a cure, and we know her cancer has a different ending planned for her than we want. So, we continually look for ways to fight her cancer, and as each day passes I am gaining more confidence and hope that Susan and I have taken some control of this thing.

For example, each day she stands out in the sun for ten to fifteen minutes to get her daily requirement of vitamin D. She meditates every day to clear her mind, and it helps to put her in a positive mental state. She does fifteen to twenty minutes of exercise daily to help keep her muscles strong and to infuse her cells with more oxygen because cancer cells don't propagate readily in a highly oxygenated environment. And, of course, she follows our new diet.

Back to this wishing her ordeal was over. When Susan and I went for her first chemo treatment, she looked like . . . well . . . Susan. Then, this week she got her third treatment. Now she looks like a cancer patient. Susan and I were waiting out in the Kaiser parking lot by the portable where she was going to have her PET scan done. She looked at me and said, "I wish this was over." And I immediately thought, whoa . . . better watch out what we wish for because "over" might mean her fight with cancer ends—it could end well or it could end badly for her.

We Are Truly Humbled
By Jeff Weaver — Apr 28, 2012, 9:19 a.m.

Yesterday was one of those days when the good and bad paid a visit to our home.

First the bad. This cycle of chemo is the worst yet. Susan is feeling the cumulative effects of the drugs. She is tired and very sick. Her bones ache, her head aches, her teeth ache, and for all I know her . . . ah . . . how to put this . . . rear end still aches from the past infection.

She was lying on the couch telling me that she was such a wuss. However, I don't buy that. There is a look in her eyes when she complains. It's not a give-in look but rather one of defiance.

Now for the good. I have thought about how to put what happened yesterday into words. How can I say what Susan felt without sounding like I am overdoing it?

I had just got home from work, and Susan was opening the mail. She had something from Macy's. She opened the letter and then broke out in tears. I sat there watching her sob, and then she wiped the tears from her eyes and said, "I don't deserve this. I feel so guilty."

She handed me the letter to read. I didn't know what to say to her.

You see, her friends and coworkers at Macy's have donated some of their hard-earned vacation days to Susan. Who does this sort of thing anyway? I don't know how we will ever be able to repay their generosity and kindness.

I told her that she shouldn't feel guilty and that her Macy's family would not do it if they didn't think she was deserving; after all, it's not like one of those corporate fund-raisers where employees feel obligated or pressured to donate. I said, "Look, they did this because you're their friend and because they feel for you and many of them truly respect you."

These donations will help pay Susan's health insurance premiums. We simply could not have paid them on our own. That means that her coworkers are playing an instrumental part in Susan's fight against her deadly disease.

We thank each of them from the bottom of our hearts.

Anniversary
By Jeff Weaver — Apr 29, 2012, 12:29 p.m.
Tomorrow Susan and I will celebrate our twenty-sixth anniversary. We are going to spend it quietly at home. Susan and I enjoy each other's company very much; in fact, I can't think of a single person I would rather hang out with. She has been my best friend as well as the one who keeps me centered. Like all couples who have spent many years together, we have had our share of fights and disagreements and disappointments, and we have hurt each other's feelings. But, for us, we have grown closer because of all the trials we have faced.

Happy anniversary, Susan. I love you.

More New Studies
By Jeff Weaver — May 3, 2012, 11:10 a.m.
I just finished reading on Fox News in the Health section about a new study that was published in the latest issue of the *Journal of Nutrition* (April 26, 2012). The Australian researchers found that "eating more corn, lentils, peas, beans and other legumes can reduce the risk of developing bowel cancer."

The study focused on the resistant starch common to these foods. Resistant starch is a type of fiber that can't be digested and that ferments as it passes through the bowels.

They suggest that eating more resistant starch "protects against DNA damage in the colon, which is what can cause cancer."

Legumes, some whole-grain breads and cereals, firm bananas, and cooked potatoes, pasta, and rice are all good sources of resistant starch.

They found that "it takes about 15 years from the first bowel cancer-initiating DNA damage to full-blown cancer, so the sooner we improve our diets the better."

Then, I found another article about the cancer-fighting properties of oregano. A study conducted by the Federation of American Societies for Experimental Biology found that carvacrol, a compound that is abundant in oregano, "is a powerful antioxidant that fights bacteria and inflammation" and can kill prostate cancer cells. Plus, it may also be effective against breast cancer cells (Fox News, April 25, 2012).

The researchers are testing a new drug containing carvacrol, and the early report is that carvacrol "is an extremely potent anti-cancer agent—eliminating nearly all the prostate cancer cells it was tested against." It was also reported that the compound stopped nearly 100 percent of cancerous cell growth.

Susan and I are on our third week with the new diet. I won't kid you, it is difficult to maintain. Not because the food tastes bad; to the contrary, it is quite good. But we are not in the habit of eating like this, and we have to plan our meals in advance as well as learn how to pair the new ingredients into complete meals. And I think the biggest part of following this diet is time, because it takes more time to cook from scratch.

To be successful with this diet, we knew we had to have a plan. Because it is a whole foods, plant-based diet, we threw out everything in the pantry and fridge that we couldn't eat, which was nearly everything. And then I made a menu, kind of like the ones we had in grade school. I wrote down what we would have for every meal for the week, and then made a list of all the ingredients needed to make each meal, and we went shopping for only those things. It made it a lot easier.

So, enjoy that whole-grain pasta or veggie pizza . . . sprinkle on a little extra oregano . . . it's good for you.

It's a Sweet Thing
By Jeff Weaver — May 7, 2012, 6:17 p.m.
We love our sweets. So much so that we, meaning you and me and the rest of us humans, consume in the neighborhood of 160,000,000 tons of the sweet stuff annually, according to the United States

Department of Agriculture (USDA).

Sugar is a crystalline carbohydrate. The main types of sugar include sucrose, fructose, glucose, and lactose.

Over the years many studies have been done about sugar and its relationship to cancer. Research indicates there's a strong connection between sugar and cancer, especially survival of cancer cells.

The research shows that tumors have altered metabolic profiles and have high rates of glucose uptake and glycolysis (a metabolic process that breaks down carbohydrates and sugars and releases energy for the body). Although these metabolic changes are not the primary defects that cause cancer, for many different types of cancer they do create the conditions needed to allow the cells to metastasize and invade. That is because the excess sugar uptake by the cells creates an environment that enables the formation of new blood vessels involved in cancer growth.

Recent molecular studies show that the multiple genetic alterations brought on by excess sugar consumption cause tumor development and direct negative affect on glycolysis. This gives tumor cells the ability to create a mass of new blood vessels.

The link between sugar and cancer can be explained by how sugar feeds cancer cells, helps them develop and then proliferate through cancer metastases.

Like us, cancer cells have a sweet tooth. They consume between ten and fifty times more glucose than surrounding healthy cells. PET scans, which detect glucose consumption, have shown that the higher the rate of glucose accumulation in cancer cells, the more aggressive the tumor. That means the tumors are more invasive and more likely to metastasize. The more rapid their proliferation, the more glucose cancer cells consume, thus robbing the healthy cells of the food they need to function correctly and even survive.

These findings suggest that controlling your blood sugar can make a substantial difference in controlling the course of cancer.

Because tumors absorb sugar at such a high rate, it is critical that people with cancer eliminate as much sugar from their diet as possible. Let me just say, as a sugar junkie myself, that this is no easy task. And there is a scientific reason why it is hard to give up sugar.

People who are addicted to smoking, alcohol, and cocaine have fewer dopamine receptors in their brains. That means the dopamine signals sent between cells are weaker, which in essence means the cells send out signals that they want more of what they are addicted to. Dopamine is the reward chemical for our brains. Well, sugar acts just like the other addictive drugs because the brain responds the same to it as to them when we eat it.

It is becoming increasingly clear to me that reducing sugar or eliminating it is one of the keys to the prevention of cancer and, more importantly for Susan, survival.

Consequently, we have become good at reading the labels on all the foods we buy. Try it yourself and compare brands and you will be surprised at how much sugar is hiding in places you would not expect to find it. Here is a helpful hint: four grams of sugar equals one teaspoon of the stuff. It takes time to shop like this, but after all, we are desperately trying to buy as much time as we can.

It seems like a fair investment to me.

Exercise and Cancer
By Jeff Weaver — May 10, 2012, 11:17 a.m.
A report was published in the *Journal of the National Cancer Institute* on the effects exercise has on cancer patients (Fox News, May 8, 2012). Being diagnosed with cancer is a terrible thing. Some cancers are easily treated, some are long-term chronic diseases, and some come with a death sentence.

The research team looked at twenty-seven different studies from 1950 to 2011 that dealt with exercise and cancer survival. They found that being physically active and exercising benefited all cancer patients by lowering insulin levels, reducing inflammation, and improving the immune system.

However, the report found that exercise had the biggest effect on breast cancer. They found that "exercise significantly reduced death from all causes including breast cancer." And concluded that "treatments may increase survival, but at a cost of quality of life; [whereas] physical activity may not only extend life but also enhances quality."

It is also important that cancer survivors know that exercise reduces the risk of recurrence up to 50 percent. And physical *inactivity* is linked to breast cancer, colon cancer, prostate cancer, and even melanoma.

So, a healthy lifestyle that includes regular exercise and a healthy diet looks to be essential for helping cancer survivors reduce the risk of recurrences as well as the incidence of many other life-threatening diseases.

But for those who are fighting cancer . . .

It is imperative they use exercise and diet as tools to buy time because the future is loaded with new and exciting treatment options.

Living with Cancer and Its Many Faces
By Jeff Weaver — May 12, 2012, 7:52 p.m.

Cancer has a face. Want to see it? Just look in the mirror and you will see one. It comes in many guises and shapes and colors and expressions.

You must be thinking I've lost my marbles. Nope. That face you see in the mirror is a face that has been affected either directly or indirectly by this disease.

When I found out Susan had cancer, I started talking to others about it. I can't recall a single person who hasn't either been diagnosed with cancer him- or herself or had a family member or close friend who has been diagnosed with cancer. It is mind boggling to me how intertwined this disease is in our lives. And depending on who has it, be it a friend or friend of a friend, a brother or sister, mother or father, son or daughter, or in my case a spouse, we are influenced by cancer in some way. And your whole life changes as a result of it.

This past Thursday was a wonderful day . . . no . . . make that, a great day. What made it so good, you ask?

Again it was the result of actions by Susan's friends and coworkers at Macy's. They had set up a fund-raiser to help with medical expenses. The deal was that if anyone took a flier in to Ruby's Diner at the Laguna Hills Mall, 20 percent of the proceeds would go to Susan. This could not have come at a better time.

It's been over two months since Susan has seen her friends. The last time they saw her only a couple of them knew what she had growing and spreading inside her, working its evil, trying to take her from us. She was "normal," just Susan. A good many of Susan's friends are signers, merchandisers, salespeople, dock workers, and managers, all working together performing the same tasks day after day. I wasn't there, but I bet when she left the store that last day no one noticed the stress and worry that showed on her face because of the news she had gotten the day before.

Today Susan isn't the same person they once knew. Every day she changes and evolves. Cancer has taken a toll on her physically, but more so emotionally. When she looks in the mirror at night, she says she sees the effects cancer has already had on her. It's taken her hair, sapped her strength, and stolen part of her future. And she sees it in the mirror's reflection. I really see it in her eyes. There is not much joy in them these days. But she is learning to live with this disease.

Susan and I got to Ruby's first, and we were seated in the back at a table with a beautiful bouquet of flowers. We never heard who did that, but we are thankful. Then her friends started showing up. They came to the back and they all hugged Susan. Big hugs. Long hugs. Joyful hugs.

I was going to take some photos, but for some reason I couldn't; all I wanted to do was sit back and watch how happy she was as she greeted her friends. I felt a warmth spread through me as each new person approached her. Most sat down at tables and ordered lunch; some stood with Susan and talked and laughed. Susan went from table to table, sitting with them and having a great time. I watched her face light up . . . revealing a renewed spirit . . . new life, and, yes, pure joy.

After everyone went back to work or home, Susan, Josh, and I walked over to the store to find her friends who couldn't make it to Ruby's. We went from floor to floor, department by department, and at each stop there were more hugs. We went to the office and she sat with her bosses, Jesus and Maria. I saw how much she missed being part of the team.

When it was time to leave, I could tell Susan was not ready to go. I think she would have stayed all day.

Her friends at Macy's are incredible. And I saw the looks of happiness and joy . . . and concern on their faces. These people are just some of the faces of cancer because each of them has been affected to some extent by Susan's cancer.

And I think they all are closer because of it. They are a huge part of her support team, and I am not sure they know just how important they are to Susan's ability to fight her cancer and—I would go so far as to say—to her very survival. Thursday they infused some much needed energy into Susan and gave her a reason to fight a little harder. I saw it in her eyes.

Yes, Thursday was a great day.

Small Steps
By Jeff Weaver — May 16, 2012, 10:34 p.m.

We had another infection scare Tuesday. It was the same problem as last time. The wound from the past surgeries hasn't healed, and the doctors had to postpone everything again until it clears up. This infection thing is a big deal and we cannot take chances.

Susan and I met with Dr. Asuncion today. Susan got a good once-over. It seems as if the big tumor in her left breast is a tiny bit smaller and has "softened" around the edges. Dr. Asuncion said one of the lymph nodes under her arm has gotten smaller.

Susan has one more treatment of Adriamycin/Cytoxan Tuesday (if everything is okay with the infection), and then she will start a new cycle of treatments targeting the cancer in her bones. Her chemo treatment and this new treatment will be back to back. It sounds like she's in for a long, tough day.

Then, the following week they are going to do another CT scan and bone scan along with other tests. The results of these tests will determine what the next chemo drug will be.

I am not sure if the news we got today is good or bad or if this is what Dr. Asuncion expected because she didn't really comment on that. But it sounds like the drugs and all the lifestyle changes we have made are working.

Just like the old saying goes: "One step at a time."

Learning to Live with Cancer: Running for Time
By Jeff Weaver — May 22, 2012, 9:34 p.m.
It's been a while since I've been inside the locker room right before a big track meet. Not just any meet—the biggest one you'll ever participate in. One for all the marbles.

I'm not the athlete this time. I am the coach working with a distance runner. Only now, as a coach, the feelings are different from when I ran. Back then, I was cocky . . . confident of the outcome . . . because it was up to me whether I won or lost. I knew deep down no one was going to beat me. Now I can only give advice and make sure my runner is prepared.

We walked down the tunnel to where the other athletes waited to hear their name called. Some sat on the benches, eyes straight ahead, focusing on their event. Some sat upright, rocking back and forth; some sat back, watching the others, or they talked to their coaches. Others paced up and down the tunnel, hoping to relax, trying to stay focused.

My runner and I sat. She looked straight ahead. I watched the others closely. One runner was walking the length of the tunnel; she stretched her arms over her head a few times or swung them behind her back. She adjusted her hat this way and that way, finally pulling it down a little tighter. Down the tunnel two experienced runners talked like old friends. They talked about techniques and what training diets they were on, and they talked about times and distances. On the other side of them, another runner looked unsettled. It wasn't her first meet, but she was still new to it all and it showed on her face and the way she wiggled her fingers. My runner sat cross-legged and wiggled her feet back and forth . . . nonstop. But they all had one thing in common: they looked like warriors.

A rookie sat down next to us. She was really nervous. She ran her fingers through her hair and asked my runner what was going to happen; she asked how she was going to feel. She wanted to know how my runner did things, what it was like for her. I was proud of my girl. She looked poised and confident, and she understood the other girl's worries. She talked to her like an old pro. My girl was ready.

Then I heard the officials start calling names. Rachel, Christopher, Kimberly, Margarita, Isabel . . . then my runner's.

We walked into the arena. The officials, dressed in blue uniforms and with badges hanging from their necks, hurried here and there. We took our place. Out came the tape: time to wrap up the runners. The officials set the timers, and then the gun sounded. . . .

Okay, so by now you know I'm not talking about a track meet. I was in the chemotherapy section of the hospital, and my runner, Susan, was there for her last cycle of A/C and the first cycle of the drug for her bones, Aredia. But it's a race nonetheless. And it's the biggest race of each of these runners' lives. And I couldn't help but notice how each person mentally prepared for their treatments, much like an athlete preparing for an event. The point is they are all in a race for time. And for some, like Susan, they are in a race *against* time because they are in a battle for their very lives. They are warriors all, combating cancer.

When the nurse stuck the needle for the IV drip into Susan's arm, Susan clenched her teeth. The look on her face is different now from the first time. There is a look of determination.

All I could do was watch and silently cheer her on. Both of us are learning how to fight. We are also learning to live with cancer.

Signs and Baby Birds

By Jeff Weaver — May 25, 2012, 12:35 p.m.

Our dining room table sits right next to a big window. If the shades are open, we can see the front yard, the driveway, and the street. But that means anyone walking down the sidewalk or driving by in a car or living across the street can see everything we do. So, these days we keep the blinds pulled. Susan does not want anyone seeing her bald head.

We didn't notice them as they built their home and moved in. I heard them now and again, but it never dawned on me that we had new neighbors. In fact, I didn't even notice them when I went outside. My mind is elsewhere these days. I've been consumed with things like diet, infections, and money.

Well, about three weeks ago I was watering my plants (I love to garden, it's therapy for me) when I first saw our new neighbors. I have a flower basket hanging outside from the eaves, in front of our dining room window. I stuck the hose up there to give my plant a good soaking. Then I started to pinch off the old flowers and a few dried twigs. I stood on my tippy toes to clean the dead leaves from the dirt, and I saw a nest made of grass and small twigs, many of them from my plant. That's when I saw them . . . four tiny baby birds.

Funny how you don't notice things that are right in front of your eyes. The world changes every minute, things come and go, and unless you keep your eyes open you can miss some very important stuff.

I had seen a couple birds landing in my basket for weeks. But I dismissed it because I thought they were eating the seeds from the dried flowers or the bugs that were on the plant. But instead they were building a home. Someplace they thought was safe enough to raise their babies.

I rushed in to tell Susan and said something like, "Hey, come over here and see what I found, a bird's nest with four brand-new babies in it. . . . You should like them, they're bald just like you." Well, maybe I didn't put it in those exact words, but close enough because I got "the look." Susan came over and stood on a chair so she could see them. She had to look closely because they were small and they blended in so well with the brown stalks and dried grass used to build the nest.

Nature is good at hiding things.

Our dining room is between the living room and the kitchen, and whenever we went from one to the other we would stop and check out the babies. We opened the window so we could see them better and kept it open. We watched as mom and dad brought them food. Susan spent a lot of time by the window, and she talked to momma bird and talked to the babies. They were too small to notice her. But they grew fast.

Susan was fascinated by those babies. As they got bigger, she spent more time over at the window, looking out at them, checking on them, worrying about them, and talking to them. As they grew bigger they would chirp as loud as they could when mom or dad came back. They opened their mouths wide, stretching their fuzzy little necks as far as they could. They knew instinctively that the louder they chirped the more food they got. As soon as mom flew off, their instincts told them to hide.

A couple weeks ago they started to grow feathers and move around a little in their small nest. It was getting crowded in there. One baby, the loudest, was getting much bigger than the others. We always knew when mom or dad was near because we could hear them. They got bolder and they were getting used to seeing Susan and hearing her voice. They stopped hiding from her. Each day they got bigger, and the loud one was venturing farther out of the nest. He would stand up and try out his new wings. He would climb up the plant so he could see his new world. And now when Susan talked to him, he would talk back to her. She got very attached to these little birds and she worried about them. And she really worried about the smallest one. It wasn't as loud or as pushy as the others.

Tuesday when we got home from her marathon chemo session, she went to the window and noticed the babies were gone, all of them, even the little one. She was afraid that something had happened to them. I went out and looked at the ground under the plant . . . no babies. . . . I walked around the yard . . . no babies. They had flown the coop, so to speak.

I went in the house and told Susan that her babies must be all right and that it was time for them to venture out into the world. She went to the window often to see if they were back. The momma and daddy bird checked in every few hours. Susan would talk to momma. But the babies didn't come back; they were gone for good.

Susan still worried. What if something had happened? she asked me. What if some big bird had eaten them? Or, if not, how would they make it on their own? Who would teach them what to eat, where to stay? Who would protect them? I told her not to worry because nature has her ways of doing things.

Last night she spent hours on the computer trying to figure out exactly what kind of birds they were. I told her I had checked earlier and I thought they might be house sparrows. She kept looking and said, no, they were house finches. It was important to her to know whether they were finches or sparrows. She told me what they ate, that they would fly to the ground under the nest first and stay there for a while before flying off, and that blue jays would eat them in the nest. She was obsessing over her babies.

Susan loved those little birds, and I have been trying to figure out why she got so attached to them. I keep wondering what the message is in this tale. Is it her motherly instincts coming out? Is she worrying so much now because she feels helpless or has no control? I can't put my finger on it, but I know it's something.

Then it dawned on me there are some parallels here and a lesson in this tale for all of us. Things happen for a reason and Mother Nature has her own way of doing things. And sometimes there's nothing we can do about the course Nature takes.

We get busy with the day-to-day things in life, and more often than not we don't notice what is happening right under our noses. Like the birds that built the nest in my plant and laid four brown and white spotted eggs and then sat on them, keeping them warm, and from those small eggs hatched baby birds that grew and grew before we noticed they were there.

If we had paid attention to the signs, we would have noticed something was up. Mother Nature will always tip her hand in some way. Like gathering storm clouds will let you know rain is coming. Then you can roll up the windows in the car or take an umbrella with you. But if you ignore the signs, well, we all know what happens.

So, slow down a little, look around, and don't ignore her signs, like the extra weight you're gaining, the pain that won't go away, the funny-looking thing on your skin, or the lump in your breast. She is speaking to you.

Oh, and one last thing. Susan made sure to let me know that finches nest twice each summer. . . . So, I'm under orders not to mess with that nest.

Rough Week
By Jeff Weaver — Jun 1, 2012, 5:00 p.m.
This has been Susan's toughest week and a half yet. That double-whammy session she had on the twenty-second has really gotten to her. Or, like they say in timber country back in Oregon, put the boots to her.

Usually, the worst days after her chemo are Thursdays through Sundays, and then she starts to feel a little better. But not this time.

To make matters worse, she had her CT scan yesterday, and so they filled her up with more wonderful things. Last night was a hard one. Today she had her PET scan done, and they put some toxic radioactive stuff in her, and undoubtedly it too will make her feel awful.

She asked me last night why she felt so bad, and then she said something must be wrong. Indeed there is. I keep telling her she has cancer . . . it has spread . . . and your doctors are filling you with toxic crap that is designed to kill the cells in you, and it has a cumulative effect.

This morning she was hurting so much she couldn't hide it. I watched her walking from the bedroom to the kitchen with her head down and eyes on the floor, her shoulders looked like she was carrying a hundred pounds, and she could barely lift her feet off the floor. I wanted to do something to make her feel better, anything at all. But there is not a darn thing I can do except to be there for her.

On a positive note, I have renewed hope. The reason for my optimism is the more I read on the effects diet has on the human body, the more I realize we might just beat this thing by starving it to death and by providing the body with the right things so her immune system can do what it is meant to do . . . kill diseases. That and Susan is good about keeping up on her exercising and getting enough sun. We are doing what we can by making significant lifestyle changes.

As I watched Susan this morning I kind of got mad at myself for ignoring some of this stuff over the years and, worse, making fun of others who chose to eat differently; it just ain't American, I thought. Well, I was right in a way. We Westerners have our own diet. Most all the studies I've read and all the research I've seen point to a sad fact: our Western diet doesn't do much in the way of disease prevention and in fact it does the opposite. So, I figure if I can provide enough information that helps just one person, it will have been worth it. I know the "I could get hit by a truck tomorrow" thing, but let me say this: when you see someone close to you so sick it makes you sick, and when you know there is not a damn thing you can do to ease her pain, and when you realize the one you love has been told she has only a few years to live, well, that does have a way of changing your tune, so to speak.

New Research and Treatments: Just Around the Corner
By Jeff Weaver — Jun 4, 2012, 12:35 p.m.

I came across a press release this morning dealing with a big national conference of more than thirty thousand cancer specialists (the American Society of Clinical Oncologists annual meeting). There is real excitement in the medical community over some of the new drugs and treatments in the war on cancer.

Here are a few highlights:
- A new class of drugs is being developed that will deliver potent drugs directly to the cancer cell and not to the healthy cells.

- A new tool has been designed to assist the immune system to attack and kill cancer cells.
- There are treatments targeting newly discovered genes and the pathways cancer uses to spread.
- The Food and Drug Administration announced it will speed up the process so that some breast cancer drugs are available faster.

Also, with the advancement in drugs and treatments, survival times are increasing. I think that this news validates part of the strategy Susan and I have implemented. Our first goal was to "buy" time until they find a medical treatment that will cure her. The second part of our strategy is to help cure her with diet.

One thing I haven't written about much here is that I am a cancer survivor. Several years ago I was diagnosed with melanoma that had metastasized. I had access to a new cutting-edge drug and an alternative treatment program. It has been over ten years, and I have only had one other brush with cancer and that was not life-threatening.

So, with the advancement in medicine and my personal experience along with diet, we remain confident that we can and will win this battle.

I Say Tomato . . . You Hear Something Else
By Jeff Weaver — Jun 8, 2012, 1:44 p.m.

This week I was reminded about the effect our words can have. And how, at times, we should be careful with our word choice and, more importantly, the message those words are conveying to others.

What I want to talk about today is what it's like being a caregiver. Susan and I have gotten dozens of messages from others who are also caregivers for loved ones. And for some, it is all consuming and extremely difficult. Being a caregiver changes your life to the point where you don't have much of a life of your own. It is stressful. You worry constantly, and you get worn down physically and emotionally.

You do it because you feel obligated or because no one else will or, as in my case, because it comes with the "in sickness and in health . . . and till death do us part" deal.

However, I'm glad I'm the one who "gets" to be Susan's caregiver. It's because I love her, and I have always thought, in part, my role has been to watch out for her and to do my best to take care of her. I'm not saying Ann and Marty wouldn't be as willing and as good at it, because they would be, but I know that with my personality I will throw my heart and soul into not only caring for her day-to-day needs but also going beyond that and doing everything I can to help cure her. Susan says one of my faults is I get too focused on things, to the point of obsessing. Well, now that fault turns to a plus.

For now, Susan needs a hand once in a while, but if she has to she can still do almost everything on her own. But for some of you who are reading this, that is not the case. You care for someone who can't manage without help and you are their lifeline. That is a lot of pressure and stress.

For being a caregiver can also mean guilt. I know I feel it. It's a "what if" thing. What if I had made sure Susan had checkups more often, what if I had picked up on the clear messages she was sending me for the past eight or nine months and made her go to the doctor, what if I had paid attention to how fatigued she was getting . . . what if . . . what if . . .

Guilt is something that eats at you, and it can make you react to others in a way you wouldn't normally. It can make you say things that may hurt others unintentionally. And that can strain your relationships with other family members or friends to the point of inflicting real damage if you are not careful.

My dad and I have a somewhat strained relationship because of some of my past actions, but usually it's okay. I love my dad, he has always been one of my heroes, and I have lived my entire life trying to please him. At sixty-three, I am still trying.

With everything Susan is going through, I sometimes forget Dad has his own set of issues. He is the caregiver for my mom, who has advanced Alzheimer's. Her memory is going very fast and most of the time she doesn't remember me or my family. It's heart breaking. Dad has taken on all her duties as well as runs the farm. He cooks and cleans and cares for Mom. He has had to alter his life in order to care for her, and it can't be easy to see the one you love and been married to for over sixty-four years go through what she is suffering from. I feel for him, and I respect how hard he is trying to provide for her needs.

This week I called him to give him an update on Susan because he doesn't read her blog, so I make sure he knows what is going on. Dad isn't much of a talker on the phone, and he doesn't hear very well either, so our conversations are a little tough to get through. I told him how Susan was doing, what the doctors told us, and then I started to tell him about our new diet. I told him we had gone to a whole foods, plant-based diet and that we had cut out meat, dairy, processed foods, sugar . . . and then I made a mistake, a big one.

I started to tell him everything I had learned about the effect a Western diet had on health and how many diseases could have been prevented by not eating certain types of foods. I told him that 70 to 90 percent of heart disease, cancer, diabetes, and Alzheimer's could have been prevented by diet.

He got angry with me and asked me pointedly if I was lecturing him. I was taken aback and a little hurt. You see, in my enthusiasm for what Susan and I are doing I wanted to share with him that we thought there is hope, that we might beat her cancer by eating differently.

I forgot he makes a living raising cows. I forgot he is living his own nightmare with Mom's Alzheimer's. I forgot about choosing my words correctly. And I forgot that what some view as great information others view as preaching or, in Dad's case, lecturing. And that is what he heard: me telling him in a roundabout way that because of the lifestyle he lives he somehow was in part responsible for Mom's Alzheimer's and that he wasn't caring for her properly now.

And I forgot how hard some caregivers have it and that I need to think about the words I say. I so wish I could take back parts of that conversation!

So, when I am writing about diet in the future or if I am talking to someone about it, I will remember this latest lesson my dad taught me: choose your words with care and try to remember how they will fall on others' ears.

A Conversation with Susan
By Jeff Weaver — Jun 10, 2012, 9:40 p.m.

This week Susan will start her next round of chemo. Tomorrow we meet with Dr. Asuncion and she will let us know how the chemo treatments did. We have our fingers crossed.

On my walk this morning, I thought about how it would be interesting to do an interview with Susan.

When I told Susan that I wanted to ask her a few questions, she gave me the "are you crazy" look. I explained to her that I thought it was important for everyone to hear from her and, more importantly, that we might be able to help others who are going through this and who can't put some of the tougher things into words.

She agreed.

Me: First thing is everyone who reads the blog probably wants to know why you don't write journal entries.

Susan: Remember, this was your idea. And at first I didn't want to share my personal problems. I'm uncomfortable with that. It's also exhausting to talk about what's going on.

Me: What about now?

Susan: It's your thing now. Besides, I'm afraid I would leave someone out. So many people have done so much . . . what if I forgot someone? I don't want to hurt anyone's feelings. Plus, most of the time I'm just not up to it.

Me: Okay. I keep you filled in on who checks in and leaves messages for you, but how often do you check in?

Susan: Since I found out you posted pictures of me (laugh) I started checking in a lot more. Maybe once or twice a week.

Me: What surprises you the most about what you read?

Susan: (long pause) Let's see. . . . I guess it's how many people post who I don't really know or know that well. And their friends and old friends of mine . . . ones I haven't seen or heard from since high school. That really surprises me.

Me: Does it help when you read their messages?

Susan: Sure, I guess I didn't realize how many people really care.

Me: So, what do you think about your friends at Macy's and what they have done?

Susan: I don't know how to put it into words. I just can't thank them enough. I can't bake them cookies either because I'm afraid I would eat them. (laugh)

Me: What about your mom? She's amazing.

Susan: Yeah . . . I think that's just Mom though. It doesn't surprise me. But what does is that so many of her friends sent cards and left messages for me.

Me: And your dad? It has to be tough for him.

Susan: He's real quiet. And I don't want to hurt him, he's been through enough . . . you know what I mean. . . . [Just a note here: Susan's brother, Ed, died in an auto wreck in 1994.]

Me: It's okay. Let's talk about how you are doing. I'm sure everyone wants to hear about that. Can you tell me how you feel physically?

Susan: Sometimes I feel like a wuss! A couple weeks ago I wanted you to shoot me. I asked Nicki to shoot me. . . . I even asked Jesus to shoot me . . . but nobody would. (laugh) I was let down by that.

Me: What's the worst part of this so far?

Susan: I'm bald!!! I'm so out of shape. I hate that, it's nasty.

Me: For me, the easy part would be the physical, but what about the mental part of this? That's something that's not very easy to see or even talk about. How are you handling everything emotionally?

Susan: It's hard. It goes back and forth, from the physical and the emotional. After the last treatment, it was bad. I'm really scared. I know it's hard on the kids because they went through this when you were sick. Now it's hard because I don't want to hurt them and I don't want to hurt Mom and Dad after what they went through with Ed . . . how much . . .

Me: I'm sorry, it's okay. . . . (pause) Okay, so we are five months into this. When you first got the news back in February, what was your biggest fear?

Susan: How much it was going to hurt the kids and you. I worried about dying, but it's not the worst thing. . . . It doesn't feel real. I mean, I don't feel like I'm dying. Then I was afraid of the chemo and the surgery. About going under anesthesia—that scares me, I'm afraid I won't wake up. We've had two pets that didn't . . . it really worries me. Now I worry about what chemo will do to me long term. I wonder if it will cause more trouble, more cancer or something.

Me: So, what about tomorrow? Are you nervous and what are you hoping for?

Susan: No, I'm not that apprehensive. I'd like to hear I'm doing better. I hope with all we're doing with the diet it's helping, because if I'm going through all this and it isn't working I'll be pissed. I worry that it will come back after the chemo is done. I can't stay on chemo my whole life. I can't take that.

Me: So, what do you think of the diet?

Susan: Like I said, if it doesn't work, I'm going to be pissed. It's hard. It's not that I don't like it . . . the food . . . but it's not . . . not normal. It's kind of a pain in the butt.

Me: Are you confident it will work?

Susan: I just don't know. You're more confident than I am.

Me: Then why are you doing it?

Susan: I gotta do something, and it can't hurt and I know it will help with some things, but . . .

Me: Okay . . . what's the hardest part, I mean, what do you miss the most?

Susan: Cupcakes, cookies, bacon, and eggs.

Me: Is there anything you would like to convey to everyone on here?

Susan: Yes: do eat healthy. I never realized how important it was before. It can't hurt you anyway. And go see the doctor even if you can't afford to. This isn't worth it. If you let your friends help you if you can't afford it, you'll be astounded at all the help you'll get.

The Grades Are In

By Jeff Weaver — Jun 11, 2012, 4:37 p.m.

Susan got the grades on her exams. She got an A+. That's right: an A damn +! Dr. Asuncion was very pleased with the test results.

So, here is what she told us. First, the scans showed no new cancer activity—anywhere. And she can't see or feel the cancerous lymph nodes in Susan's armpits. The tumors in Susan's right breast have shrunk significantly. And the biggest tumor that is in her left breast shows improvement as well.

The best news is that Susan is going to get a break from the chemo. Dr. Asuncion wants Susan to be completely healed from the surgery she had due to the infection. So, no chemo. She is going on an estrogen therapy treatment. Tomorrow instead of the Taxol she will get an injection of Faslodex along with the Aredia treatment for her bones. She will have six Faslodex injections and then be reevaluated.

Susan will sit down with her surgeon, Dr. Luby, to see whether she is going to do the surgery before Susan has to go back on chemo.

So, what do you think Susan's first question to Dr. Asuncion was? "Does this mean my hair will grow back?"

The answer: "Yes, but—"

Susan interrupted her and said, "That means it's going to fall out again, doesn't it?"

Dr. Asuncion smiled and said, "Well, keep your hair short. This will just be a tease."

And for me the best news is, I don't have to give Susan those nightly shots. I do hate those. And maybe, just maybe, she can eat salads and fresh tomatoes and have some lettuce on her veggie tacos.

Good news and small steps. But, at the end of the day, Susan still is a stage 4 breast cancer patient. She still has active tumors in her breasts, active areas in the lungs, and maybe the most worrisome is the cancer in her bones.

It's a long way to the finish line.

New News
By Jeff Weaver — Jun 12, 2012, 10:22 p.m.

Yesterday, as soon as we got home, Susan got a call from Dr. Luby, her surgeon. The doctor wanted to see us today and told Susan her treatments had been moved to next Tuesday. I was thinking, well, that was quick.

This morning we met with Dr. Luby, and we didn't know if she was going to tell us she would do the double mastectomy or not do it. Yesterday there was still some uncertainty because, as we were told before, the mastectomy wouldn't do much in the way of prolonging Susan's life because the cancer in her lymph system and lungs and bones would get her before the breast tumors would. However, Dr. Luby and Dr. Asuncion had had a pow-wow.

When Dr. Luby came into the exam room, she sat down in front of the computer. She explained that Dr. Asuncion was so pleased with what she saw that she believed it was time to rethink and review all options. Dr. Luby had not looked at the scans or the official analysis, so she pulled up Susan's chart and read. The first word out of her mouth was "*Wow*." She was genuinely surprised and quite happy. As Dr. Luby read the chart, both Susan and I read it as well. I read that there was no trace of live cancer in the lymph system and that the cancer in the lung area was barely visible.

She told us that things were different now and that she wanted to do a double mastectomy, remove the tumors in Susan's breast, especially the one that has grown into the chest wall, and take out the lymph nodes under her arms. By doing this, she said, we might have a slim chance of beating it or at the very least buy more time and hopefully in the future there would be some new treatments that would be able to cure her cancer.

I can't tell you how ecstatic I was. But then I'm not a woman. Apparently, you women place a higher priority on hair and boobs than even life itself because the look on Susan's face was like this was the worst possible news she could have gotten. I know she said she was afraid of going under anesthesia, but what was going through my mind was, we're talking about your life here, baby, so whatever it takes, let's get it done.

On the ride home we talked about the mastectomy at length. I assured her I didn't give one whit about her boobs. (I tried to say that tactfully because I know I was on thin ice with that kind of talk.) She tried to compare her boobs to my . . . well . . . boys. I'm thinking, no, and had a killer counter as to why that comparison was way off base, but I thought better of it, so I asked her whether she wanted to increase her chance of survival or not.

So, after much thinking and an argument or two, Susan decided she's having the surgery. Most likely in two or three weeks.

What surprises me is how well Susan is doing. In all the reading and the research I've done, I know the progress she has made is nearly unheard of in such a short time period. Her doctors also think the same thing. I think we owe this success to Susan's doctors, the drugs, and people's prayers. And I am convinced the diet and other lifestyle changes have played a major role in this turnaround. I know from my competitive days in athletics and my Army days that the best and most surefire way to win a battle is to prepare, train, study tactics, find your opponent's weakness, and attack on all fronts, never faltering in the heat of the battle. I feel like that is exactly what Susan and I are doing.

Now, excuse me while I go do some research on the importance of boobs to women in the modern era. I have a lot to learn. But just between you and me—I truly don't give a darn about her boobs; I just want to grow old with Susan, with or without boobs.

Problems for Cancer Survivors
By Jeff Weaver — Jun 14, 2012, 1:26 p.m.

Most doctors outside the oncology community have never learned what the impact cancer treatments may have on the longer lifespans they fight to achieve for their patients.

According to the National Cancer Institute, this can mean big problems for the thousands of cancer survivors in the United States, and the number of survivors is growing every year as a result of new drugs and earlier detection.

Inside the cancer community it is known that some of the long-term problems come from the chemotherapy drugs that have been and still are used to treat cancer. For example, Adriamycin can affect heart function, and many patients who have taken this drug have experienced heart failure. Many times, the problems with their heart come without prior warning or any symptoms. But the biggest problem is once patients finish chemotherapy treatments the oncologist sends them back to their family doctor. This can be a real problem for cancer patients, one that potentially puts them at great risk.

I read an article on Reuters about the American Society of Clinical Oncology meeting last week (June 5, 2012). Members were presented the results of a large survey of primary care doctors, internists, and family practitioners on the long-term side effects of common chemotherapy drugs used in the treatment of breast cancer and prostate cancer.

Turns out that 94 percent of those surveyed did not know about the side effects, which include heart problems as well as "osteoporosis, nerve damage, early menopause, infertility, leukemia and the recurrence of cancer."

The article also points out that most insurance plans cover oncology visits for a limited time, and then the patient has to return to the primary care doctor. But that can lead to issues if the oncology doctors don't share information and provide the family doctor information on the drugs that were used and their long-term side effects.

Even more worrisome is that only a third of the oncologists knew what the long-term side effects of chemotherapy treatments were.

With the recent good news Susan received, I am starting to think about what kind of side effects she will have to deal with in the future because of her chemotherapy treatments and radiation treatments.

It is never too early to start planning and to understand just what she will be up against. The more we know about what she has been treated with will allow us to make smarter decisions in regard to her health and the health care she will receive in the future.

I know many of you have gone through your own battle with cancer, and unfortunately many of you will go through it in the future. I hope providing this kind of information helps in some small way.

Information is a powerful thing.

Learning to Live with Cancer: A Different Kind of Father's Day
By Jeff Weaver — Jun 18, 2012, 12:58 a.m.

Today is Father's Day. I am blessed with two awesome children and two step-children, so I know today is going to be a great day.

It is starting to heat up down here in So Cal. I got up early, and Mick and I went for our usual four-mile walk because he can't take the heat as well as I can, and frankly, I can't take it like I used to. And hot weather really bothers Susan. She is dealing with chemo-induced menopause and the awful hot flashes that come with it. We are learning to plan our days now.

Nothing is the same as it used to be. But this morning I thought I could escape all that for a little while. You see, Josh is taking me to an Angels game this afternoon. Our beloved Angels are playing the Arizona Diamondbacks. Nicki is coming over to spend the day with Susan . . . just like the old days when Josh and I would go off for a day of father-son fun and the girls would do . . . well, whatever girls do.

After my walk, the plan was for Susan and I to go do our weekly grocery shopping. As I finished reading the paper, I noticed something was bothering her. I've gotten into the habit of watching her pretty closely. I noticed she was near tears. I saw her wipe her eyes. She looked troubled. I waited for this to pass, but it didn't, so I asked her what was bothering her. She wouldn't tell me. After several gentle attempts, I let it go. But we didn't go shopping.

When it comes to Susan, not much escapes me. I know when she hurts, when she is feeling better, and lately I am watching for the times when she is mentally down. One of the side effects of chemo is depression.

One thing I am working on is giving her more space, not hovering over her so much. It is hard for me. And I think maybe for most men because by nature we are "fixers." We see a problem, we want to fix it. It's what we do; it's what makes us feel needed and useful. But there are things we can't fix.

Around eleven fifteen Josh came out of his room with the tickets and a card. He said, "Happy Father's Day," and waited for me to open the card. I knew it would have some sort of body function joke in it because for us boys some of these functions are always funny no matter how many times we see or hear them. I was not disappointed.

Before we left I gave Susan the shopping list. I thought maybe it would be good for her to go out on her own. She has only gone out a couple of times by herself since she was diagnosed. I kissed her, and off Josh and I went. I was excited. I love going to the Angels games. And I needed the break. I was getting tired physically and mentally from dealing with her cancer, too. I thought being out in the sun at the ballpark, surrounded by Angels fans, and all the other things that go with being at the ballpark would be just the ticket.

On the way there I told Josh something was really bothering Mom. I told him I didn't know what it was, but I thought maybe it was the surgery next week, that it must be the thought of having her boobs removed that was so upsetting to her. He agreed. We talked about the surgery for most of the way to the stadium . . . not our usual banter. I don't think we mentioned batting averages, who was pitching, or what wondrous caloric vein-plugging food we wanted to try. God, I love ballpark food!

We got to the game, and people were tailgating everywhere. Smoke was coming off the grills as ribs and burgers and dogs and corn on the cob and anything you can shove a stick through cooked. Kids were running around dressed in red Angels jerseys with the names of Weaver (not ours, but Jared Weaver), Pujols, Hunter, Trout, and other players on the back. Fathers had on their jerseys too and cold beer next to the grills. It was going to be a great day for a game—I could feel it in the air.

Inside the park Josh led me to our seats. And, man, what seats!

Section 102, row B, seats 5 and 6. Just two rows back from the four-foot-high fence that separated us from the players. I love the pregame stuff and the singing of the anthem (I always tear up if it's done right, and that day it was), and I love the sights and sounds in the stands. Usually, that is.

But today some loud-mouthed guy sat right behind us. He was in his forties or early fifties. His daughters brought him to the game. He was one of those people who tries too hard to be cool. His language was inappropriate for all the little kids around. He invaded everyone's space, including mine. He actually put his arm around me and jammed a rally monkey into the side of my head. My patience with things is sorely lacking these days. I am constantly on the verge of losing my temper, so I have to be careful not to snap at people. Josh leaned over and reminded me that every time we go to a game there is some jerk nearby and told me to ignore the guy. He was right. Still, I wanted to tear that puppet off the man's hand and stuff it up his . . . well, you know, but I took Josh's advice. I did, however, turn around and stare a hole right through him. I think Josh was relieved that was all I did.

One thing I noticed today that bothered me was all the sugary treats the kids were eating. Cotton candy and ice cream, red vines and Cracker Jacks (yup, they still sell them), and Cokes. After all, it was a day at the ballpark. Families having fun. But what I saw was kids eating themselves into future health issues. I kind of wanted to say something to the parents, but frankly it's none of my business.

It was hot, but a breeze blew through the stadium just enough to make it nice. The game was good, a pitchers' duel, and then Pujols hit a monster shot into the centerfield bleachers. Everyone jumped to their feet and the stadium rocked; lights flashed all around and fireworks exploded in the blue sky over the waterfalls. It dawned on me that I was still in my seat. All I could think of was Susan and how I would rather be home with her. I think Josh felt it, too, because he didn't get as excited and vocal as he usually does. Don't get me wrong, I did enjoy the game. And I loved being there with Josh.

But today it just wasn't the same.

When we got home Nicki was there and she had a gift for me: an Oregon Duck Gnome. He is cute. I love gnomes, and sadly I have quite a collection of them. Susan, Nicki, and I cooked dinner. Then we all sat at the table and ate, just as we have on so many other Sundays. It has always been a big deal at our home. We talked about the diet. And we talked about what Susan can and can't eat and why. We talked about the evils of sugar and other no-no's on her list. We talked about the surgery. These are the new topics at the dinner table, and they weigh a lot more than the old topics.

Susan gave me a card, and I opened it and read it. It was beautiful. She always picks the best cards and this one nearly made me cry.

After Nicki got in her car and went home, Susan and I stood out in the yard. The breeze was soft and brought in the much-appreciated cool air from the ocean. I gave Susan a big hug, right there where the neighbors could see. We held each other tight and I told her I loved her.

Back in the house, Josh was in his room, and it was just me and Susan. But we were not alone.

We live everyday now with cancer, and it permeates each thread in the fabric of our lives with its stench and its deadly threat. It hangs over us like a dark storm cloud and it has changed how we look at everything. It makes it hard to fully enjoy things we used to relish, like red vines and hotdogs and sunny days at the game, and time around the dinner table with our children.

Learning to Live with Cancer: Scars
By Jeff Weaver — Jun 21, 2012, 9:45 p.m.
I wrote a short story a while back and one of the lines is "You can tell a lot about people if you just look. Life leaves marks." The story is about a man with a big scar on his face, but it really is about the many different kinds of scars you get in life. And what kind of mark you leave behind.

Life is a strange game sometimes. Last week we were ecstatic. Today . . . not so much. You would think at my age I would know the deal by now: sometimes you take one step forward, then it's back to Go. Victories are, as they say, fleeting because the next challenge is just around the corner.

Next week Susan has her surgery. Today we had her pre-op meeting. As I mentioned earlier, Susan is not only dreading this surgery because she fears going under anesthesia and the knife. I know something else is bothering her, but I don't know what it is.

I have also mentioned on several occasions that I feel helpless at times and it tears my insides apart because there are things I just can't fix for her. When I went through my own battle with cancer, I kept most everything from her because I didn't want her to worry or get stressed. It was easy to do because I was up in Mill Valley all week and only home on the weekends. I thought I was protecting her. But now how do I do that? How can I tell her everything is going to be all right? The truth is, I can't.

The stress and tension levels have been rising as we get closer to the surgery. We have been told by many that this is a piece of cake. Don't worry, they say, everything will be fine, and eventually she will look better than ever. No doubt there is truth in those words. It does help, and she truly appreciates the words of encouragement.

The ride down to Irvine was quiet. The music on the radio was so low we could hardly hear it. We didn't speak more than a few words. When we got to the hospital, she checked in and we went up to the surgical floor and sat in a waiting room. I could see the stress plastered across her face. I made a couple stupid jokes about things (I can't even remember about what now), trying to break the tension. It didn't work.

Before the PA came in, Susan couldn't hold it in anymore. She started to cry. She told me she didn't want to do this. I said something stupid again, and again I don't even remember what I said. She started to laugh a little and threatened to beat me. But the tears were still there, and all I could do was say more empty words, trying to make her feel better.

Craig, the PA, finally appeared. He is the same man we saw at the very start of Susan's battle. He is in his fifties and a big man, but he is also caring and gentle. It shows in his movements and in his voice. It's not an act. I wondered how many times he has done this. How many people, like Susan, who are fighting for their lives has he counseled and had to explain what they were about to do? And how many times has he had to calm them when he asks for their signature on the consent forms? I don't think I want his job.

Craig is very good at explaining everything. He asked us if we had any questions for him or for Dr. Luby. He went over the consent forms with Susan and started to hand them to her. Susan said, "I don't want to do this," and broke out in tears again. She tried to apologize and said she was having a little meltdown.

I sat there, watching her cry. I saw how terrified she was. It was all I could do to hold back my own tears. In fact, I didn't, but she couldn't see them through her own.

On the drive back home, both of us were in a somber mood. No joking around. No music. We were mostly silent. I can't tell you what Susan was thinking about. Me, I was still trying to hold in my tears. I was very close to having my own meltdown. But I was also trying to contain my growing anger.

Susan is afraid of the surgery, but I think a big part of her fear is that it is another reminder that this is some serious stuff she is dealing with. Everything she goes through reminds her that she has cancer and doesn't have much control and her life could end a lot sooner than she ever thought.

And the surgery is going to take part of her womanhood from her, part of her identity, leaving behind nothing but scars. And that, I think, is part of what Susan fears the most.

I hate this damn disease. I hate what it is doing to Susan, to her parents, to the kids. I hate that it has altered our lives in such a dramatic way. I am angry that I can't take it from her and beat the living snot out of it, and then kill it with my bare hands.

No matter what happens, we all will be horribly scarred by it.

Like I wrote in my story: "Life leaves marks." And "you can tell a lot about people if you just look."

When I look at Susan, I see a brave and courageous woman who is now terrified. But one thing I am certain about is, I will always see the beautiful girl I fell in love with.

Chicken Soup and Mom
By Jeff Weaver — Jun 24, 2012, 2:21 p.m.
Once in my writing workshop I read aloud the first draft of a story I had written about a man and his relationship with his two children. When I finished reading, my professor, Lisa Alvarez, said matter-of-factly, "You like to write about relationships." I was a little surprised, but she was right. Most of the stories I write are not about some incident or event, but about how people interact with one another. The main theme is always about the personal and emotional dynamics of those relationships.

I was thinking about that on my walk this morning. I thought about my relationship with my children. Once Susan told me—well, more like scolded me—that I treated Nicole and Josh differently and that I was harder on Josh. She was right. I do treat them differently. I tried to tell her that my job as a dad was to get each of them ready to take on the world and help them survive and hopefully prosper. I said dads are harder on their sons than they are on their daughters. I'm not sure I made my point though.

That's because she is a mother. And we all know that the relationship with our moms is different from the one with our dads. The old axiom about men being from Mars and women from Venus also holds true with mothers and fathers. We are different. A lot different.

Think about this for a minute. How many times have you tuned in to a sporting event and at the end the victorious athlete looks at the camera and says, "Hi, Mom"? It's rarely "Hi, Dad." On battlefields throughout history the last words of dying soldiers are to their mothers. When youngsters fall off a bike and skin a knee or cut a lip, they run to mom. When you were young, who was the parent who comforted you, sat at your side, and ran their hand through your hair? Whose words were always softer and carried some kind of magical power? Who made you that special meal when you were down? I'm sure many dads do these things, but usually it's mom.

Susan is busy cleaning the house. She is a little stressed but also excited. That's because Susan's mom, Ann, is coming down to help out after Susan has her surgery. She will be here sometime tomorrow if she can navigate LA traffic. I've been to Brookings, Oregon; it's a lot different here.

I'm looking forward to the help as well. But I'm looking forward to something else, something much more important. Something I can't do for Susan and something I can't give her.

My words don't carry the same magic as a mother's words do. And God knows that Susan can sure use a little dose of that old mom magic.

Like when we were young and had a bad cold and mom would bring us a hot bowl of chicken soup. I can hear the words now . . .

"Here, eat some of this, it will make it all better."

An Emotional Couple Days
By Jeff Weaver — Jun 27, 2012, 11:07 a.m.
Most of us have some sort of phobia; mine is needles and shots. I hate them. I fear them and have since I was little. I still break out in the sweats when I have to get one. Irrational . . . stupid . . . yes . . . but for the life of me, I can't get over it.

Susan is terrified at the thought of going under anesthesia. The fear that something could go wrong during surgery is another part of it. She knows it can happen. My uncle Ray went into the hospital several years ago for a simple day procedure and he never came home, and she thinks of that. So, I know when I get home from work tonight I am going to need to be careful of what I say. It's good Ann is here. That helps.

8:45 p.m.: We had a wonderful surprise tonight. Lisa and Francesca came over to see Susan. They are her friends from Macy's and the two "instigators" who raised all of the money for her. They got here just in time for dinner. So, they got to try one of my go-to dishes on our diet: Lemony Minty Lentils, and fruit smoothies.

They came into the house and Susan introduced them to her

mom. Then, Francesca handed Susan something. She said, "I hope you like it. We didn't know what to do for you and so we did this." Susan took the bag and pulled out a blanket. They had had all Susan's friends at work write messages and sign it for her.

After dinner Susan, Ann, and the girls sat at the table and talked. When I finished cleaning up, I went into the living room and watched them. They were laughing, sharing work stories with each other, and they talked about their families. Then the topic turned to tomorrow and the surgery.

There was a shift in their moods. I could see Susan's eyes start to turn red. I knew she was struggling to hold in her tears. It didn't work. She said to them, "I don't wanna do this." That's all it took. She burst out in tears. I watched Francesca, and she looked like she wanted to do something to help (and cry at the same time). But what? I mean, what can any of us do to help Susan get through this besides offering our hugs, a few words, and our love?

When Lisa and Francesca were ready to leave, we all walked out to Francesca's car. There were hugs aplenty. Susan has a special place in her heart for Francesca. She is like a daughter to Susan. When they hugged it was easy to see the genuine love they have for each other. And, yes, I started to cry. I had to turn around and take a few steps back. I didn't want Susan seeing me be so weak when I'm telling her she has to be strong.

My emotions are all over the place. Susan may be holding up better than I am. Just a second ago I almost picked up this stupid computer and threw it out the window. My word processing program is all messed up and I have no patience for this kind of crap.

The house is quiet now. Susan is getting ready for bed, Ann is petting the dogs, Josh is in his room, and I am finishing up this part of the journal. And Susan still has cancer and she is dreading tomorrow. It's going to be a long night, I fear.

The Surgery
By Jeff Weaver — Jun 28, 2012, 7:30 p.m.
I didn't sleep a wink last night. Neither did Susan. I got up to feed

the dogs and took my shower. Ann was up early, and Susan was right behind her. We had to leave the house by seven to make sure we would be at the hospital by eight thirty.

Susan and I went in one car, and Josh and Ann came down later. When we checked in at the nurse's station, Susan was asked the same questions for the thousandth time: Can I see your ID to make sure you are who you say you are? (Seriously, they ask that.) Do you still live here? Are you allergic to anything? And on and on.

Then she had to sign the consent form again, and she choked up and cried again. The nurse asked Susan if she could pray for her. Susan said yes, because by now she is used to people saying, "I'll pray for you." What Susan didn't realize was that the nurse meant right now and reached out and took her hand and prayed aloud for her. I noticed the others in the line behind her bowed their heads as well.

Well, that got me. I started crying . . . again. And, yes, I feel like a dope for crying so much and for writing it down, but that's just how it is now. All this surprised Susan and she was uncomfortable with it. When she came over and sat down, she asked me why people do that. I told her, "It's because they believe it will help." After a short pause I told her, "And it will help if you believe too."

Nicole got there right after Susan and I. She brought some vegan chocolate cookies. I told Susan she could have some when she got out of surgery. Before Josh and Ann arrived, around nine, they called Susan into pre-op.

We got a number and we could check where in the process she was by watching an electronic message board. 180565 . . . in pre-op, 180565 . . . prepping for surgery, and so on. I think this is weird but at the same time helpful.

Finally, a nurse came out and told us we could go back and sit with Susan before they took her into the operating room, but only two at a time. So, we took turns. Nicole and I went back first. When Nicole left to go get Josh for his turn, she gave Susan a fist bump. The surgery was supposed to be at ten thirty, but we had to wait until eleven forty-five when they finally came to give her the sedative shot and took her away. This extra time just added to Susan's stress!

I stood there and watched as they wheeled her bed through the pre-op room. The nurses dressed in their blue gowns, blue hairnets on, blue sacks over their shoes. Susan tried to look back, but she was so tied up in tubes and cords that she couldn't turn her head far enough. The last thing I saw was the big white hairnet she had on that made her look far older than she is and a purple sock with a dog paw on it sticking out from the end of her rolling bed.

One thing I know for sure: the Susan I saw being rolled into surgery isn't going to be the same one I will see when she gets through. She is always going to carry the scars left by cancer.

At 2:10 Dr. Luby came out to speak to us. She told us the surgery went well. But she found three more suspicious lymph nodes that they had not seen before, and she was pretty sure they were cancerous, so she removed them. My worry meter went way up. She told us we would know next week what the biopsy found. For now, we are all just thankful the surgery went well.

Dr. Luby said it would be about an hour before Susan came to, so we waited for Susan to wake up. Up on the board I saw 180565 in Recovery 2.

One hour turned to one and a half hours, but finally a nurse came out of the door leading to the recovery room and asked for the Weaver family. I looked around and the four of us perked up. I thought, "Damn straight, lady, . . . we are one hell of a family." Just like before, only two of us were allowed to go back at a time. Nicole and Ann went first.

It wasn't but a few minutes and I heard my name. Nicole was at the door calling me. She said I needed to go back to the recovery room because the nurse wanted to go over the procedures for Susan's post-op care. So, I joined Ann because we would be the ones caring for Susan.

The nurse, Jennifer, showed us how to empty the plastic collection bottles taped to Susan's chest. They are collecting the blood from the drain tubes that are inserted into the ends of the incision. Apparently, we need to measure how much fluid comes out and document it on a chart. We were told to check the tubes for clots and make sure to check for signs of infection around the incisions as well as the place where the drain tubes are inserted into Susan's chest.

When Jennifer opened the gown covering Susan, I was taken aback. I have seen many wounds in my time, and I've seen severely injured people, but this really got to me. And it wasn't like I didn't know what was coming. The impact of seeing my wife lying there looking so delicate and in so much pain with a big fresh wound from one side of her chest to the other was . . . well, more than I bargained for. I suddenly felt like throwing up. And it wasn't from the wounds as much as from seeing Susan like that. Even writing this, I'm having a tough time maintaining my composure, and containing my anger.

I looked over at Ann, and she too was struggling with the sight of her only daughter lying there with tubes coming out of her chest and that big fresh wound still bleeding. My God, what must have been going through her mind.

Finally, at five thirty we got the okay from Dr. Luby that we could take Susan home.

It took us over an hour to get from Irvine to Diamond Bar. Rush hour traffic up I-5 is always a bear this time of day, but the 57 freeway is worse. First thing we did when we got home was make sure Susan took a couple of pain pills. The last thing we needed was for the pain meds to wear off. We were told she was going to be in considerable pain.

Josh and I got Susan all settled in. Then Ann and I put ice packs on her chest. It was soon time to empty the collection bottles. We were in for another sleepless night. Thank God Ann is here and for Josh and Nicole. I didn't think I could do this by myself and give Susan everything she needed.

Recovery
By Jeff Weaver — Jul 6, 2012, 6:45 p.m.

It has been a crazy and very busy few days. Susan is finally starting to feel a little better. Not so much intense pain and she is moving around better, too.

Ann and I both hated dumping those blood-filled collection bottles and messing with the bandages, but that has thankfully come to an end. We are all very tired, and I can't wait until we get back the routine we had before the surgery. As bad as that is sometimes, it is a hell of a lot better than the past several days.

Susan and Ann are doing a lot of catching up, and I am taking advantage of some extra time to catch up at work. This is really affecting my income.

Looks like Ann might be leaving soon. I know that will be hard for Susan when her mom does head back to Brookings. I have to say I am proud of Ann. She is one hell of a mother, and maybe the best mother-in-law ever.

Learning to Live with Cancer: The Roads We Travel
By Jeff Weaver — Jul 8, 2012, 4:47 p.m.

Each of us travels different roads. Today Ann's travels will take her to San Rafael to visit a friend. Tomorrow she will make her way up the 101 to Santa Rosa to see Alix, Susan's aunt, then on to Brookings. To home and to Martin, to her everyday life. But it is my guess her life will not be the same.

It has been two weeks since Ann arrived at our home. She came to help Susan after her surgery. And help she did, but in ways she may not know.

Susan's road since February has been one filled with far too many obstacles. And not enough carefree moments or moments filled with laughter. For a short time Ann provided some of that, and in so doing she lifted Susan up mentally.

Ann left shortly after eight this morning. We said our goodbyes and of course there were tears when Susan and Ann put their arms around each other. Our house will be awfully quiet without her here.

And Now We Fight

A short while after Ann left, I forced myself to go on my walk even though I wasn't really in the mood. But I couldn't seem to walk at my normal fast pace. Even Mick seemed to be dragging a little. We just didn't have any energy.

On my walk I go through a nice neighborhood, filled with well-kept homes. The streets are lined with palm, sycamore, pine, and California pepper trees. As I walked, all I could think about was Susan and what she must be feeling now that her mother was gone. I have been trying to hold my emotions in check while Ann was here, but I couldn't do it any longer. I sat down on a low stone wall under a pine tree, buried my face in my hands, and sobbed like some hormonal thirteen-year-old. For the life of me, I couldn't stop crying.

Then I heard someone ask if I was all right. I couldn't answer, and a woman's voice asked again. I felt her hand on my shoulder. I looked up and it was the lady I see every Sunday out walking her dog. We always wave to one another and say good morning as we pass. I told her I was okay, that I was just worried about my wife. She looked at the pink band I wear on my wrist. She seemed to understand, nodded, and headed on her way.

I finally collected myself and resumed my walk. I headed down the hill toward home. Mick was worried about me and stayed right by my side, looking up at me the rest of the way.

Josh sees his mom every day, and he is affected a lot more than he lets on. He holds everything in and pretends that life is pretty much normal. It is not, and I hope he is doing okay.

Nicole is our rock. She has helped us more than I can say here. She has sacrificed more than any twenty-four-year-old should have to and put her own plans on hold. Her road has taken a hard turn.

My road is now one of a caregiver. I rarely think of anything but my wife. Well, I always did that but in a totally different way if you know what I mean. Now it's how can I help her live longer and make what time she has better? I hope that I don't let Ann and Marty down. I hope that I will see the day when Susan and Nicki and Ann can spend the day doing things without the burden and weight of cancer hanging over them. And most of all, I hope that someday I can hold my wife in my arms, look into her eyes, and see that sparkle that makes her special rather than the tears that remind me that we still have a very difficult journey ahead of us.

And for Susan, her road always leads back to this: she is the one who has cancer and she has to live with the pain, the treatments, the fear, and the fact she doesn't know who will win the battle she is fighting every single day.

New Doctor, New Plan
By Jeff Weaver — Jul 14, 2012, 12:34 p.m.
Jesus told his disciples a parable to show them that they should always pray and not give up.
—Luke 18:1

Carol Davis sent Susan *Streams in the Desert*. It's a book of daily devotional readings. I read it every night. I came across this passage and the message with it: "The failure to persevere is the most common problem in prayer and intercession. We begin to pray for something, raising our petitions for the day, the week, or even the month, but then if we have not received a definite answer, we quickly give up." It goes on to say, "Giving up is admitting failure and defeat."

As I've said, I believe strongly in the power of prayer; in fact, I believe that prayer amplified by many voices is a powerful force.

I also believe that we all need help at one time or another in life. Without help, few of us would make it. Having a strong support system is one key to success. I can't imagine where we would be without Ann and Marty, the Macy's crew, Josh, Nicole, David, Lisa, Francesca, all the doctors Susan has seen, and all the other people who have supported her.

But there's more to it than that. We all must do everything in our power to succeed, to thrive, or sometimes even to survive.

Susan is not a quitter. But I truly think she would not have heard what she did yesterday without the prayers and support from those who have logged in and left messages, offered prayers, raised money, sent cards, called, visited, offered diet tips, and many other acts of kindness and, at times, personal sacrifice.

We may be witnessing a medical miracle, my friends.

It is the only thing I can think of that explains what we were told by her new oncologist. Dr. Kashani is one of the most respected and experienced oncologists in the area. So, when he said he couldn't believe what he saw, it was surprising but very exciting. After he reviewed Susan's charts and test results, he said it was amazing how far she has come in such a short time period. He said that her newest test results show no new activity! He couldn't stop talking about the incredible progress Susan was making. He used the word *miracle*.

But the best news was this: he is thinking of changing the plan from one of extending her life to one of curing her. He thinks we now have a shot at beating this.

In the next couple of weeks, Susan will meet with the radiologists to set up a schedule for radiation treatments. We want to make sure there is not a single ember of cancer that could reignite at a later time.

We told Dr. Kashani about all the changes we've made to our diet and why and about the other lifestyle changes, and he was surprised that we have made so many changes, but he was genuinely pleased—I think maybe more that we are so dedicated and determined than for any other reason. He told us it is rare that cancer patients do what we have done.

Susan and I fully understand that this is great news. I am personally elated that Dr. Kashani is so amazed at how well Susan is doing. It means we are doing something right. Susan and I talked about this on the way home and I ask her if she was excited. Her answer surprised me a little. She said, "Not really. Dr. Asuncion has been telling me she was so happy about how I'm doing. But I don't want to get my hopes up too much either, because she always said I would probably have to go through all this again." And that is a stark reminder that she is far from being done with this fight. Cancer has a nasty habit of popping up again if you let your guard down, even for a little while. So, we promise to keep our end of the bargain and fight like heck.

The Legend of Senbazuru
By Jeff Weaver — Jul 16, 2012, 9:22 p.m.

When I first saw it hanging from the dining room ceiling, I told Susan it looked like a piñata. And I thought that was rather appropriate because Susan and I feel like we've been beaten with a stick a few too many times lately.

But then Susan asked me to come take a closer look. I asked her what it was. She said it is a Japanese origami made up of a thousand handmade folded paper cranes (*Senbazuru* in Japanese). She said it was a gift that Yoko, her friend and coworker from Macy's, had made for her.

In case you aren't familiar with origami cranes, they play a part in an ancient Japanese legend that promises that anyone who folds a thousand origami cranes will be granted one wish, commonly long life or recovery from an illness. It's also said that hanging them in your home is a powerful and benevolent charm.

There is a popular nonfiction story, *Sadako and the Thousand Paper Cranes*, about a girl, Sadako Sasaki, who was two years old when Hiroshima was bombed during World War II, and shortly thereafter she developed leukemia. When she was twelve, inspired by the legend of the paper cranes, she started making her own. The most popular version of this story says she got to 644 cranes before she died. But her friends, the story goes, finished the rest in her honor.

I intend to read the story this week.

Along with the origami was a beautiful card. When Susan read it to me she had to stop because she couldn't finish it. Here's what Yoko wrote:

Hi Susan, I made this thousand origami paper crane wishing you a recovery. Our legend promises that anyone who folds a thousand origami cranes will be granted a wish by a crane. So my wish has to be granted. Take good care of yourself. With lots of love, Yoko.

In Western countries the gift of origami cranes is often given to cancer patients. Susan and I will do everything to make sure Yoko's wish comes true.

I mean, how can we fail with so many prayers and wishes from so many people.

We are once again humbled.

A Letter for Susan
By Jeff Weaver — Jul 25, 2012, 5:58 p.m.
I am really trying to understand what it must be like to have a radical double mastectomy.

Susan is struggling mightily with this and more. She gets depressed and angry, she questions whether she should have had the surgery, she feels like she has made a mistake, and she even wonders whether it would have been better to keep her boobs, tumors and all, and not look like, as she says, "a freak and hideous."

I don't know what to tell her; I don't know how to help her understand what others think. So, I thought the best thing I could do is write her a letter.

Dear Susan,
I wish I could put into words exactly how I feel about you. I wish I could help you understand what I see when I look at you. I wish you knew how I feel when you hold my hand or brush against me or touch me. How can I explain the pain I feel for you and the sorrow I feel because your life has been altered so much? How can I make you know just how much I love you?

I looked in the mirror yesterday and stared at my reflection. I tried to see what you must see now. I wondered if you still see the young, fit, rugged man you met. Or do you see the gray hair, the dark circles under my eyes, the deep lines etched across my face, the sagging skin and wrinkles? Do you notice that the fire I once had for life has died down and the big dreams I once had for us are gone from my eyes?

One of my biggest fears has been that one day you will wake up and see an old broken man rather than your man. You are so much younger than I am, and I've long worried that some young, handsome man would steal you from me and I would be helpless to stop him.

After staring at myself in the mirror, I went out to the living room and sat across from you and looked at you while you napped. What I saw was a beautiful woman. I saw the woman I want to spend all the days of my life with. I saw my mate and my life partner. Like I wrote in a poem, "We've seen the hurt and the sacrifice and compromise turn to understanding. We've raised a family, shared laughter, shed tears, we've been marred, been tarnished by the wear of everyday life, but that's all right."

And because of those things I cannot imagine my life without you.

I pray every day that you will always be with me. I pray for your health and your well-being. And I pray that you understand that no matter what you've gone through it only deepens my love.

When I see you now, my respect and love for you grow by the hour. I see your strength and how hard you are fighting for your life. I see how much you love our children. I see how much you care for your parents and friends and how much they care for you. And I see your fear and I know you feel helpless and vulnerable.

Even though I will never really know and understand how you feel about what you have gone through . . . I promise you this:

You will always be my girl. Till death do us part, and I pray that day is many, many years away. I love you for who you are and what you are with all my heart.

Cancer-Detecting Dogs and a Young Scientist
By Jeff Weaver — Jul 28, 2012, 2:27 p.m.

My mailman is afraid of my dog. Mick barks at him when he leaves the mail in the box by the front door. But Mick has never tried to bite him or jump on the door to get to him. He might lick him, given the chance, but never would he bite the poor man. So, the mailman's fear is irrational. Mick is only doing what he thinks is his job, being an early warning system; heck, he barks at me when I come in the front door.

So, why do I bring this up? Because the mailman failed to deliver a certified letter from Kaiser to me. He wouldn't even knock on the door to let us know he had the letter.

Susan had to go across town to the post office to pick it up. It was a letter pleading with me to go get a colonoscopy because one of the four samples I sent to the lab (FIT test) came back positive, meaning there was blood in the stool sample.

I know I should get the colonoscopy, but I don't want to because the way this procedure is done freaks me out. And I've read about the risks. In fact, according to a large study done by the American Society for Gastrointestinal Endoscopy, 33 percent of those who undergo the procedure "have some complication" and 3 percent have a "serious adverse event," which can lead to death.

Of all people, you would think that I would be first in line, right? Wrong!

Look, with all the new technology out there today, there has to be a better way than to knock me out with anesthesia and shove a camera up my, well, you know what, all the way to my Adam's apple. It is such an invasive procedure.

Colonoscopies aren't the only cancer screening tests that are invasive. Other types of cancers need to have biopsies done. With breast cancer, they use needles to get tissue samples, while other types of cancer require surgery. All carry some degree of risk. But what if my dog could warn me with a high degree of accuracy if something was wrong? That might convince me to get the procedure done because I trust my dog.

As Susan and I look back, Jessie, our red Aussie, tried to tell her something wasn't right, but we didn't understand what she was trying to tell us. As I mentioned before, I promised Susan I wouldn't give all the details about what Jessie did, so I'm going to tell you about some research being done with dogs that can detect cancer and about a few people whose pets detected their cancer. Like they say in the movies, I changed the names to protect the innocent, and me.

Linda found out she had breast cancer after her dog discovered it by sniffing her chest. Her spaniel, Penny, had been sniffing and nuzzling at the area where an aggressive tumor was growing until Linda finally went to see her doctor. She had tests done, and the biopsies came back positive.

Maureen's collie-cross, Max, started sniffing her breath and nudging her right breast. After she got tested, nothing turned up, but Max kept bugging her. So, Maureen insisted that her doctors take another look. It turned out she had a tiny but aggressive cancerous tumor developing that doctors had failed to detect in the earlier test.

Marie, a seemingly healthy young mother, said her dog, Jazz, wouldn't leave her side. She said her dog laid her head on her feet and wrapped her front legs around her legs like she was hugging her. Whenever Marie went out, the dog would lie at the door, waiting for her to return. Jazz stood in front of her, blocking her path when she tried leaving the house, and when she went into the bathroom, the dog insisted on going in with her and would get upset when Marie, well . . . peed. A few months later Marie felt a lump in her breast and was diagnosed with cancer that had metastasized.

A group of cancer researchers in the United States tested cancer-sniffing dogs in double-blind tests (neither the dog handlers nor the experimenters knew which person had cancer and which did not). A small percentage of the test subjects had cancerous tumors, and the dogs accurately found every person with cancer. The big surprise came when the dogs pointed out three researchers. Turns out all three of them tested positive for cancer.

Several studies have tested the effectiveness of dogs' abilities to smell cancer in humans. Makes sense, right? Dogs are used to detect bombs and drugs and find people buried under snow or collapsed buildings.

I found an article in *Psychology Today,* "Mr. Dog: Medicine's Best Friend," about cancer-sniffing dogs (April 29, 2012). A Japanese study in 2011 compared how accurate a Labrador retriever was when trained to detect colorectal cancer by smelling breath and stool samples compared to colonoscopies. With breath samples, the dog was 95 percent accurate, and it was 98 percent accurate using stool samples. The researchers discovered that the dog was very effective at finding "early-stage cancer," and it was able to tell the differences between polyps and malignancies. A colonoscopy cannot do that.

In a study done in 2004, dogs "consistently identified" a sample from a healthy subject as positive for cancer, so the sample was tested again at the hospital. Finally, researchers discovered cancer on the person's kidney and bladder cancer.

In 2006, California researchers trained three Labrador retrievers and two Portuguese water dogs to detect cancer. Patients with known lung and breast cancer provided breath samples used for training the dogs. After the dogs completed their training, they were able to correctly identify 99 percent of the samples from different lung cancer patients. With breast cancer, the dogs were 88 percent accurate, with no false positives. And the dogs also identified three test volunteers who didn't know they had cancer.

There are so many stories like this it makes me wonder how many people would be saved if more effort was put into this type of noninvasive detection.

Given how effective trained cancer-sniffing dogs are, if we had better access to them, maybe people like me who are afraid of traditional cancer screening tests could go see a trained cancer-detecting dog and wouldn't have to have unnecessary and risky surgeries, biopsies, and colonoscopies, unless, of course, the dogs tell us we smell like cancer. We all have irrational fears, but for most of us, being sniffed by a warm, cuddly dog isn't one of them.

So, if Mick starts nuzzling my backside or sniffing my pee . . . you can be damned sure I'll schedule that colonoscopy.

The Ups and Downs of Cancer
By Jeff Weaver — Aug 1, 2012, 10:08 p.m.
Not too long ago I said this cancer thing is a strange game: it's one step forward, then it's back to Go. Sometimes the news from our doctors lifts our spirits to incredible heights, gives us so much hope and belief that we can overcome anything that cancer throws our

way, and then sometimes the news deflates us so fast we wonder if we can get back up again.

For the past three years I have studied words. They are, at times, incredibly powerful and can elicit laughter or tears; they can inspire or discourage. And a single word or phrase can speak volumes. So, I'm learning to be careful how I use them in certain situations. I sometimes forget that not everyone is as careful with word choice as I am.

Susan and I met with Dr. Kim today to go over her radiation treatments. Frankly, I did not like what I heard. And when we left we were confused and deflated.

Dr. Kim is a really nice guy and, I'm sure, a wonderful doctor. He is also very cautious and overexplains things. I am thinking he may do that because English isn't his native language.

As he was going over Susan's medical history with us, he used the words "stage four cancer" far more times than Susan or I cared to hear. He also said, "because we can't cure this," so many times it was discouraging.

He was going over the risks and the pluses and minuses of radiation therapy with us. He wanted to know what we wanted to do. Susan asked him what I thought was a great question: "What would you do if I was your mother?" His answer, "Well, if you were my sister I would wait, because . . . " (*Sister* is not a typo.)

This is where the conversation took the unexpected and unwelcome turn. Basically, he said because Susan is stage 4 cancer and there is no cure for her cancer, he did not want to subject her to radiation. He added that there was only a 20 to 25 percent chance the cancer would return to breast tissue where the tumors were found. He "hoped" they got all the cancerous cells cut out, but it was "on the outside margins," and if the cancer returns, they can always operate again and then do radiation.

Then the bombshell words.

"Because you have cancer in the lymph nodes in your chest and the cancer is in your bones, that's what will kill you even if the cancer returns to the original site. And I don't think you are done with chemotherapy yet, so let's see what happens after that."

We drove thirty-five miles down to Sand Canyon Hospital to find out the schedule for her treatments and where they would be administered. It seems to me that if they (Dr. Kashani, Dr. Luby, and Dr. Kim) had decided against radiation, a simple phone call saying so would have been sufficient. That aside, what caught my attention was this:

"You only have a twenty-five percent chance of the cancer returning to the original site"—as if that was remote enough not to worry about it. It's like telling me there is only one bullet in this four-shot revolver, so go ahead and point it at your head and pull the trigger. No worries. I reminded him Susan does have a small chance to beat this now, so why take the risk of allowing the cancer to return? We didn't get a clear response to that, and I was so upset I didn't press the issue.

I am worried. Susan and I would rather be proactive than reactive. We STRONGLY believe she is going to beat this because she has great doctors (even if I'm a little confused by them at times) and because of all the difficult lifestyle changes we've made.

Look, I'm probably overreacting here, so the next thing I am going to do is write a long email to Susan's oncologist—who just two weeks ago was amazed at her progress and wanted to slam the door shut on her cancer—and get some much needed clarification. As I told Dr. Kim, "You're the expert, so we are going to trust your judgment."

I think Dr. Kim doesn't understand the power and the weight his words carry and how they can either take us higher or take the air right out of our sails.

But you all can be assured that I am going to remind Dr. Kashani that we want to be aggressive with Susan's treatments because we want her cancer cured, not just managed.

We are going to kick this crap's ass . . . whatever it takes.

Learning to Live with Cancer: A Special Recipe
By Jeff Weaver — Aug 6, 2012, 5:04 p.m.

Ever wonder why someone becomes one of those special people in your life? I was thinking about that after Susan got a picture of Francesca holding her own fund-raiser for Susan by selling homemade cupcakes and cookies at a big neighborhood yard and garage sale. I wondered, why these two? Susan is as old as Francesca's mom. What was it that brought them together, and what created the bond they have?

We all know that if you want to bake a great cake, you follow a recipe. Flour, eggs, butter, milk, baking powder, salt, vanilla, and if you want a really good cake . . . chocolate. But the best cakes—the ones you marvel at—all have that one secret ingredient that makes them special.

One of the things I have tried to do here is convey what it's like to live with cancer. Not just for Susan but also for her family and friends. So, I decided to talk to Francesca and find out how this has affected her, why she has such a bond with Susan, and why she has done so much for her.

A conversation with Francesca:

JW: So, how did you first meet Susan?

FC: At work. I was working in the Swim Shop at Macy's. It's not part of the main store, it's a little shop out in the mall, and I was out there by myself. Susan would come in to check the displays and the racks to make sure the merchandise was where it should be, priced correctly, and fill in where needed. I would ask her questions, and she always took the time to answer and help me. Then we started talking about other things, personal things. She reminded me a lot of my mom.

JW: I know she considers you part of our family. She calls you her second daughter. What sort of things did you two discuss?

FC: Susan and I have always been close and have a special bond . . . a connection. I can't explain why, all I know is that it's there and I would do anything for her.

Whenever I had a problem and needed someone to talk to, she

was there for me. About two years ago I found out that my parents were moving to New Jersey. They asked me to go with them since I was only working part time and wouldn't be able to afford to live in California by myself. I was panicking. I wasn't ready to make such a drastic life change. I had nowhere to go. Then I called Susan and told her what was going on. I asked her if I could stay with her until I figured out what I was going to do. Without hesitation she invited me into her home. I remember thanking her repeatedly, and she said, "Don't worry, we won't let anything happen to you." I can't describe the feeling of relief I felt after that moment, and I will never forget that day. Anyway, from then on I considered Susan my mom.

JW: For me, what makes Susan so special is her spirit and how spunky she is. Tell me, if you can, what is it that makes her special to you?

FC: I love that she's not afraid to tell you how she feels and how she always speaks her mind. I look up to her so much because of this. She doesn't mold to what other people want her to be. She is always "Susan." I know that times haven't always been easy for you guys . . . the constant moving around, and you not working for the best employers, and you battling your own sickness.

JW: What went through your mind when she told you she had cancer?

FC: I remember the day she told me she was sick. She sent me a text asking if she could call me. This was a very unusual text from her, so I knew something was up, but I was not prepared for what she was about to tell me. She said she wouldn't be working at Macy's for a long time. When I heard this I was angry. I thought for some strange reason she had been fired. I asked her why. She said, "I have cancer." When she said that, her voice started to shake. My heart sank. I didn't want to ask too many questions because I knew how hard it was for her to make this phone call. Susan is a very private person, but she said that she thought of me as family and wanted me to hear it from her instead of someone from work. I asked her if she needed anything, someone to drive her to appointments or take her home after chemotherapy. She said she had it covered. I then told her that she's a strong person and can handle anything and beat this. She said I hope so and laughed. I said I love you and talk to you soon. She said, "I love you, too," and her voice started to shake again.

I tried to keep it together until I got off the phone. As soon as I hung up, I put my hand over my mouth and cried.

JW: You've done so much for her. How did that start?

FC: She's been through so much already. I started to think of ways I could help, so I researched "how to help a friend with cancer." What questions to ask, what questions not to ask, and how to be supportive. I knew she would be going crazy sitting at home, so I bought her the *Hunger Games* series of books and baked her cookies and treats. Then I found out that she needed to be on a special diet. So, I looked up online what foods help fight cancer and also what tasted good to patients having chemo treatments. Chicken pot pie seemed to be the answer, so I made her homemade chicken pot pie and sent it home to her along with aromatherapy stress relief bubble bath and bath salts. But then I found out how strict her new diet needed to be. This news killed me because I felt like I couldn't help her now. I was too afraid to make her anything in fear of giving her something that would hurt her. Cooking for her was my way of showing her how much I love her and am always thinking of her.

JW: So, what do you think of the diet now?

FC: Like I said, it kills me that she has to be so strict because it's one more thing I can't do for her. (Had to pause here; both of us got pretty emotional.)

I think it's a good idea. It opened my eyes. Now I try to eat better and get Ryan to. (Ryan is Francesca's long-time boyfriend.)

JW: I remember she was excited that you were coming over that night before her operation, but she was also nervous because of the way she looked. I felt a certain nervous tension as we ate. How did seeing her make you feel?

FC: Susan started to look uncomfortable and then she finally said,

"I'm really hot. Can I please take off my hat?" We said, "Yes, take it off!" She looked at us and made us promise not to freak out. I didn't know how I would react to what I saw. When she took off her hat, I was shocked at how beautiful she looked and I could still see my Susan.

JW: When you guys left, it was very emotional and I can still see you and her hugging. How did you feel then?

FC: When we were leaving, the look on her face broke my heart. She talked about the surgery and what she had to do to prepare for it. Her eyes started watering, and I could feel mine starting, too. But before I came up, a friend of mine told me not to cry, to be strong for her. When Susan finished telling us what she had to do before surgery, she looked at me, smiled, and said, "Want to go for me?" and I said I would. I meant that from the bottom of my heart.

JW: And after the surgery?

FC: I could tell Susan was feeling a little down when we were texting each other back and forth. I told her I wanted to come visit her. She said, "I don't want you to see me like this." I couldn't believe what she was saying and I didn't know how to respond. How do you tell someone what they mean to you?

So, I told her, "You are an amazing wife, mother, and friend. I love that you have moved so much over the years; Oregon, Vegas, and now California. Sometimes I feel like I'm stuck in a routine. I wanna travel and try new things, but then I'm also scared. I hope my husband loves me as much as Jeff loves you. The way you two look at each other isn't around that much these days. And I hope I'm as close with my daughter as you are with Nicki. You have always been there for me when I needed someone to talk to. I look up to you so much. You're my mom and dearest friend."

Soon after that I had the opportunity to have a bake sale for Susan. My friend's neighborhood has a huge garage sale and his mom sells eggrolls. People go crazy for them, so I was gonna sell cupcakes and cookies to raise money for Susan. I was up two nights in a row cooking until two thirty in the morning for the bake sale. About halfway in, I started to get nervous. What if nobody buys anything?

But I tried to stay positive. The next morning I set up my tables and prayed that I would sell something for her. It was such an emotional day.

So many people came up to my table asking about Susan and her story and said they would pray for her. One lady gave me twenty dollars and didn't even take anything. I said thank you so much, it really means a lot. She said, "Yes, I know, my mother also has breast cancer." When she walked away, I had to go inside because I couldn't stop crying. It was so moving that a stranger would give that much. She didn't know me or Susan and still cared enough to give us a big donation. It seemed big to me since I was only selling things for fifty cents.

When I first found out about Susan being sick, I thought about what if she was taken from us? And I would cry just thinking that. But then I had a dream two months ago and Susan was in it. I walked up to her and asked her how she felt, and she said, "I'm good, my cancer is gone." I was so excited and happy and gave her a huge hug and then I woke up. It doesn't seem like that big of a deal, but it was the feeling inside me after I woke up. The next day I called her and told her about it. And I said you're going to beat this, I have a good feeling.

JW: I'm doing this for Susan because I know how she feels about you. Anything else that you want to say?

FC: Susan makes me want to be a better person. I'm starting to figure out what I want to do in life. I want to help people like her.

I wish all the time that I could do something or give her something from my body that would take this away from her. But I can't.

So, now I dream about the day we will celebrate, when she is cured.

If you aren't moved by this conversation, please check your pulse. I know this is a long entry, but I just couldn't edit it down.

I don't know the exact recipe for friendships like Francesca and Susan's, but if I had to guess, it would go something like this:

Start with some kindness, add a heaping handful of trust, toss in some understanding, some humor and laughter, don't be afraid to add frankness, a healthy dose of truth and honesty, and don't forget to add who you really are. And for the special ingredient . . . well, each of us has our own secret sauce for that.

How May I Help You?
By Jeff Weaver — Aug 12, 2012, 9:16 p.m.

Every day at work when I answer the phone, I say, "How may I help you?" I say it so many times it is automatic.

For a long time I have felt like I am supposed to do something significant before my time here on Earth is done. But what and when and for whom? I have talked to several of my professors at school about why I'm going back to college at my age. They tell me I have the wisdom and experiences that only time gives. They say . . . teach.

In my corporate communications business, we represent publicly traded companies and we do investor relations for these small and exciting young companies. One of the cool things about my job is that I get to speak to hundreds of investment advisors and analysts from all across the country and some in other countries. The downside is that we don't receive any compensation for one to two years. Last week I took a call, and as I always do I said, "How may I help you?" I take hundreds of calls, but this one was amazing.

When Susan was diagnosed in February, I told Tony, a gentleman I speak with frequently, about it. He said his wife is also a stage 4 breast cancer patient. He told me in the last year and a half she has battled her cancer that she has had three rounds of chemo, a double mastectomy, and radiation. They were told there wasn't much hope.

A couple months later I shared with Tony what I had learned about diet and told him what Susan and I were doing. I recommended the video *Forks Over Knives* and several websites where he could read about studies on diet and cancer.

Then yesterday I got an email from Tony:

Jeff, I don't know how to thank you. When you first told me about your wife and what you were doing, Marilyn and I were desperate and we didn't know what we were going to do. I had looked into other treatment options, but they were so expensive and our insurance didn't cover them. I went to the websites you told me about and read the research about the relationship with food and cancer. I bought the video and we decided to make the change to the whole food, plant-based diet.

This week Marilyn got the results of her CT scans. We received wonderful news. Her markers are way down and the scan showed no new cancer activity. Her doctors think she may actually be close to remission.

Of course the doctors patted themselves on the back for how well the drugs worked, but I don't think that was it, because the cancer was still going strong until we changed the way we ate. I didn't argue with them because they seemed dismissive of the diet when we told them about it. Marilyn's doctor told her not to worry about that sort of thing because there was no cure, so make sure she enjoyed herself.

I know one thing for sure, we aren't changing what we are doing, and now I actually believe Marilyn has a chance. But the best part is she believes she can beat this now.

I'll talk to you Monday. Your friend, Tony.

Doesn't his story sound much like Susan's? I don't understand why doctors don't embrace diet as part of the treatment. Not to makes no medical sense whatsoever. The research is there and the numbers don't lie: 70 to 95 percent of all cancers, heart disease, and diabetes can be prevented with diet, and certain foods are known cancer killers.

I know for a fact the new diet has helped me. The excruciating pain that I have been living with in my joints due to arthritis is nearly gone. Two years ago I had a complete blood workup done and the test results showed I was at the high end of the ranges. Two weeks ago I had severe chest pains, so I went to the ER. The doctors ordered a CT scan and a complete blood workup. The scans showed no tumors in my chest. And the results of the blood test showed that my numbers were now at or below the lowest numbers in the ranges. My blood pressure is now excellent and I've lost twenty-three pounds!

For a few weeks I have had a feeling inside that I need to make one more life change. Susan and I have talked about whether I should look into studying nutrition rather than economics. I love to write, and I am continuing my education in writing this fall (I have a long way to go before I can call myself a writer). We actually talked about writing a cookbook for cancer patients. Every day, one thing is becoming clearer: I want to help educate people about the relationship they have with food and how food may, in fact, be the best medicine of all.

I can't wait to talk to Tony tomorrow. And when I say, "How may I help you?" I'll have a new appreciation for those words, a smile on my face, and a reason to study harder.

Learning to Life with Cancer: Just a Little Sweetener
By *Jeff Weaver* — Aug 20, 2012, 12:18 a.m.

Big Manny is my friend. And I worry about him. I met Manny at work three years ago, and it didn't take long for me to become friends with Manny because he is smart . . . really smart. I'm not sure there is a topic that Manny can't talk about with some authority. I call him Big Manny because he is really overweight.

Surely, he understands the risks of being overweight.

Last night Manny called. He wanted to check in and see how Susan was doing. Susan loves Manny, even though she has yet to meet him. I talk to her about him frequently. They trade barbs back and forth through me. She used to bake him cookies and I would leave them as little surprises on his desk. So, when he called I gave Susan my phone so he could hear from her how she is doing.

Manny told her he was praying for her and that he had decided to change his eating habits because of her and that he is losing weight as a result.

On my walk this morning, I was thinking about Manny and Susan. And how what Susan is going through and the changes she has made while fighting for her life have affected those around her. It's like the ripples from a single drop of rain that falls on the surface of a still pool of water. That one raindrop sends dozens of waves out in ever-widening circles, and they touch everything in the pool.

After Susan was diagnosed and when I started looking into diet, I told Manny all the things I learned. I remember telling him the most important thing he could do is cut out sugar. He's not the only one I have given that advice to. I tell anyone who will listen or who is interested in how to eat for health.

If you only do one thing, cut out as much sugar as possible and anything that turns to sugar in the body. Plus, limit foods made from processed wheat flour and white rice because they act like refined sugar when you eat them. I know it isn't easy; in fact, it's really hard and it takes willpower and time and effort, but it really is that important. Why?·

Because sugar is one of the main causes of inflammation in our cells, and inflammation is one of the root causes of so many diseases, with cancer at the top of that list, along with heart disease and diabetes. Sugar is the leading culprit in the fattening of Americans. Studies now show that body fat, especially around the middle, causes inflammation in our cells.

You have to read every label on every package of food you buy. If the ingredient list says sugar or fructose or honey or brown sugar or molasses, or any number of other sweeteners, don't buy it. We have learned to distinguish between processed sugars (which we can't eat) and naturally occurring sugars (some of which we can).

There is a big difference between refined sugars and the sugars that are in plants and fruits. The sugars in fruits and vegetables act differently in the body from how refined sugar is processed because it takes the body longer to extract the sugars. So, what are some alternatives if you want to sweeten foods and drinks?

Well, I did some reading and found a number of new studies show that some natural sweeteners are safe to consume and have less of the bad effects of processed sugars on our bodies. Then I double-checked the glycemic index of these natural sweeteners.

The **glycemic index (GI)** indicates how rapidly a carbohydrate is digested and released as sugar into the bloodstream, which affects blood glucose levels. Carbohydrates with a low GI value, 55 or less, are more slowly digested, absorbed, and metabolized, so our blood glucose and insulin levels rise more slowly.

The **glycemic load (GL)** is a little different in that it is a ranking system that measures the amount of carbohydrates in a serving of food. Foods with a GL of under 10 are considered low and will have little impact on blood sugar levels.

The glycemic index does not take into account the amount of carbohydrates in a food. So, glycemic load is a far better indicator of how a food will affect blood sugar levels.

Here are a couple of natural sweetener alternatives:

Coconut palm sugar, GI 35, GL 3. It looks and tastes like brown sugar and has a nutritional content far richer than all other commercially available sweeteners. Coconut sugar is high in potassium, magnesium, zinc, and iron and is a natural source of the vitamins B1, B2, B3, B6, and C. It is a 100 percent organic, unprocessed, unfiltered, and unbleached natural sweetener and contains no preservatives.

100 percent organic cactus agave nectar, light, GI 11, GL 1. Make sure it is 100 percent natural because many suppliers mix in other sweeteners to cut costs and still label it as "pure" agave. It is low on the glycemic index and even lower on the GL index. The light is milder than dark agave and about 1½ times sweeter than sugar, so you use less. It's best used to sweeten drinks and baked goods and in most places you use sugar.

Stevia, GI 0, GL 0. It's the best of all the natural sweeteners. It is actually a herb that does not raise your insulin levels. Stevia is one of the most health-restoring plants on Earth. It is native to Paraguay. It is a small green plant, and the leaves are used to make the sweetener we buy. It is about 30 times sweeter than sugar. Stevia leaves contain proteins, fiber, carbohydrates, iron, phosphorus, calcium, potassium, sodium, magnesium, zinc, rutin (a flavonoid), true vitamin A, and vitamin C, plus an oil that contains 53 other compounds. This zero-calorie natural sweetener does not raise blood sugar levels.

Even though Susan needs to eliminate sugar, for most other people, if you can cut back on sugar usage by substituting natural alternatives for refined sugar, you will have more energy for longer periods of time, lose weight, look better, feel better, reduce inflammation in your cells, plus reduce your chances of developing cancer, heart disease, and diabetes and live a longer and healthier life.

Susan, like that tiny drop of rain, is only one person among billions, yet her ripples are touching so many others, like Francesca and Marilyn and my friend . . . Big Manny.

Now that's a sweet thing.

A Glorious Weekend
By Jeff Weaver — Aug 27, 2012, 1:57 p.m.
It was a great weekend. So, what made it great? Let's start with boobs. Susan has been playing phone tag for a couple weeks with Macy's and Nordstrom, trying to coordinate a time so she can get her "new" boobs. Well, Saturday was the day. We went in to the lingerie department at the Nordstrom store in Brea, and while Susan and the coordinator did their thing, I sat in a comfy couch they had and waited for over an hour.

I found out a couple things while I sat and waited just a few feet from the register. One, women who shop at Nordstrom like buying small, "fancy" things no matter their age, size, or shape. Two, they didn't even give me a second look as they held up those tiny lacy garments and other girlie items. Being the gentleman I am, I averted my eyes as much as possible. Three, I was, I'm sure, a lot more self-conscious and uncomfortable than they were.

When Susan and Marta (the coordinator) finished the fitting and all the paperwork, I noticed a smile I hadn't seen in some time on Susan's face. And I saw a renewed confidence in her. I thought what a difference $676 silicon molds shaped like a woman's breasts make. On the way out, we took the escalator down to the first floor. Susan turned to me and, with her patented mischievous smile, she said, "Wanna feel my boobs?" And I did . . . right there in Nordstrom in front of hundreds of moms and teens doing their back-to-school shopping.

Slowly but surely my Susan is returning.

Speaking of returning, Susan is rehabbing everyday now, doing exercises to strengthen her upper body. She is planning her return to work. We aren't sure when, but we hope fairly soon. We meet with her oncologist on the seventh, and based on the latest test results, he will tell us what and when her treatments will be.

As we headed home, Susan and I were upbeat. She was cracking jokes, and we were laughing.

Sunday was even better.

We had planned on making dinner for Francesca, Nicki, and Kevin. I wanted to show Francesca how to make a few healthy and tasty meals. Susan and I went grocery shopping early. Then we did some of the prep work for the menu. I made appetizers: spicy, savory, roasted chickpeas and roasted sweet potato rounds.

When Nicki and Kevin arrived, Nicki wanted to help in the kitchen, so she and Susan went to work preparing ingredients and I started cooking. Nicki invited Courtney, her childhood best friend, to join us. Courtney and Nicki met when we moved to Las Vegas in 1997, and they've been best friends since. After we moved here, Courtney moved over here a couple years later. Courtney is like Nikos (Josh's best friend) and Francesca, one of our "other kids."

Francesca arrived next. Soon our home was filled with our family . . . and laughter and the smell of food cooking. Everyone was helping.

The girls and Kevin sat down, and Susan and I started serving. Veggie pizza (except for Kev's pepperoni pizza, he doesn't do veggies . . . yet), a brown rice noodle dish with spinach, peppers, cucumbers, and peaches, and Francesca's fave, minty lemony lentils. I also made an avocado kale salad, and we had lots of different kinds of fresh fruit.

We ate, we talked, we laughed. We had a blast. I could see the pride in Susan's eyes. And I could see the love she has for all her kids.

When the conversation turned to Susan's cancer, there was a more upbeat and confident tone. Everyone, including Susan, was happy and filled with hope. We talked about the future and a time when cancer wouldn't be the center of attention.

Around eight thirty everyone had to leave. But it took a long time for them to say their goodbyes. Of course there were plenty of hugs.

But one thing was missing this time: the tears.

Paying It Forward
By Jeff Weaver — Aug 31, 2012, 2:50 p.m.

The days are getting a little shorter now. Susan and I are getting busier. It seems, for me at least, there just isn't enough time in the day for me to do what I need to. And that worries me a little on a couple of fronts.

My work is taking up ten hours a day. This has reduced the time I have in the evening to cook. My education resumed last week, and after just two class sessions I know I'm in for a long, tough semester. One of my professors is a young, brilliant woman from my mom's hometown, Binghamton, New York. The expectations she has for her students are high. If I'm to succeed, that means hours of writing and lots of reading. It is exciting in a way because she will push me farther than I have ever been pushed in my writing. But it means even less time, and that is my biggest concern.

Cooking for Susan is one of the most important things I can do for her. And she is the single most important thing in my life, so I need to learn to manage my time better and come up with ways to cook that are less time consuming.

That got me thinking about other people. Everyone has busy lives these days, and not many of you want to spend extra time planning menus and cooking from scratch and what I call close shopping. Close shopping is reading labels and understanding what is in the food you buy and what these ingredients do to you. It is a must-have skill if you want to eat for health and, for some like Susan, for life itself.

Susan and I are making plans for the future—well, more like plans for the near future. I came up with an idea a couple weeks ago and ran it by several friends and colleagues. As I've said before, there is a huge hole in the treatment plans most cancer patients receive: information on diet. With all the studies that have proved beyond a doubt that diet may be one of the most important aspects in the cure and prevention of cancer, it makes absolutely no sense that this subject is nearly ignored.

My idea is to write a cookbook for cancer patients. This will combine my newfound love of writing and my need to help Susan beat her disease and my long-held belief that I have some other purpose in life. It's a project that Susan and I can do together. I think this could be a great resource for people who are diagnosed with cancer. Most people don't realize that eating the right foods could help prolong their lives . . . and maybe even beat their disease. And most of the so-called cancer cookbooks I've seen are more geared for making meals that are easy to prepare or they come up short when the goal is to use food as a treatment. In fact, I haven't found one where every single ingredient fights cancer and where foods are paired so as to get the maximum benefit from the cancer-fighting compounds.

Susan and I know how hard it is to figure out how to eat like we do now, and we also know how important it is. So, why not share our knowledge with others? Make life a little easier for other cancer patients at a time when their lives are turned upside down.

The cookbook will be filled with great-tasting recipes made with cancer-fighting ingredients and nothing in the food that aids tumor growth or damages a person's cells. And we'd mix in short pieces on what the ingredients do for a cancer patient and how they fight cancer as well as include short, simple-to-understand pieces on new research on the relationship between food and cancer.

I think it is important to include all that, because when people understand why and how something really works they are more apt to start and stick with it.

That brings me back to Susan and me. Lately, I have been letting her down. I noticed that I haven't been as strict with her foods as I should be. I haven't taken the time to plan all her meals carefully and pair the foods for maximum effect. I haven't been loading them up with the best cancer-fighting ingredients. When we got the great news about her progress, we breathed a sigh of relief and I think I took my foot off the gas a little. That is unacceptable.

Because we have been given so much help from others, this is a way that Susan and I can pay it forward, by giving others hope, by optimizing their chances of living longer and richer lives, and maybe even by helping them in some small way beat the odds.

Thinner Is Better
By Jeff Weaver — Sep 6, 2012, 4:35 p.m.
One thing we might add to Susan's diet is a little salmon. Everything I've read indicates that the benefits (known cancer-fighting proteins and nutrients) outweigh the risks (mostly toxins from polluted waters). About the only thing I can find objectionable about salmon is where it is caught and how. I don't worry about the how—that's for the animal rights folks to debate—but I do care where. Salmon caught in Alaska or the Northern Atlantic live in much less polluted waters and are safe to eat because they aren't loaded down with toxins.

A big plus is salmon helps with weight loss. It's those omega-3 fatty acids.

This morning I ran across a new study on body fat and cancer.

For some reason many Americans don't think or seem to care that carrying extra pounds is a big health risk. But here is the reality: being obese can take twenty years off your life. And as I have noted before, belly fat greatly increases the risk of cancer, especially breast cancer.

Obese sounds like really fat people, right? Not so. Just last year, according to all the charts I read, I was considered obese. My BMI (body mass index) said so. I was 232 pounds and at 6 foot 3 inches, everyone said I was thin. Take a look at any chart online to find your BMI; it might surprise you.

But here is the good news. Losing even a small amount of weight can reduce and sometimes reverse the risks.

A recent study from the University of Texas MD Anderson Cancer Center found that overweight women have four times the endometrial cancer risk (cancer of the lining of the uterus), and for the same reason they're at increased risk for breast cancer: body fat produces estrogen, which is linked to both types of cancers. Additionally, University of Minnesota researchers found that leptin, a hormone associated with weight gain, increased the production of breast cancer cells.

Obese people, particularly those with belly fat at midlife, are 260 percent more likely to develop dementia. And the bigger the belly, the greater the risk, because of hormones or inflammatory factors produced by the abdominal fat. There is that word again: *inflammation*.

Just a side note here: researchers from Kaiser Permanente found that people with the fattest arms at ages forty to forty-five were 59 percent more likely to have dementia later in life.

Another finding is that obese women have a higher risk of complications from breast reconstruction after a mastectomy. What's worse is that they also are less likely than normal-weight women to get the full benefit of presurgery chemotherapy, mainly because doctors worry about toxicity from the drugs, so they tend to give overweight women smaller doses than they really need because they know the toxins are stored in their fat cells.

And let's not forget about the connection between being overweight and heart disease and diabetes.

All this proves to me that Susan and I made a wise choice by changing our diet. We are fighting and hopefully winning the battle with her cancer, and as of this morning I was down to 191 pounds from 232 when we started eating for health. That's 41 pounds since March. Last week I had to buy new jeans, a 34-inch waist—something I haven't seen since I met Susan in 1985!

I can't emphasize this enough: eating better is a smart way to manage your health by managing your weight, and it may spare you or someone you love from hearing . . .

"I'm so sorry, you have cancer."

Short Medical Update
By Jeff Weaver — Sep 8, 2012, 1:07 p.m.
Yesterday Susan and I met with Dr. Kashani for a progress report.

First thing, he reiterated his desire to be aggressive going forward because of the progress Susan is making. So, she is going to stay on the Faslodex, Aredia, and Lupron.

We asked him how long will she be on these drugs. He told us the Lupron is short term; however, the Faslodex and Aredia may be for a very long time unless something changes—like, she goes into full remission; then maybe she can stop or if, God forbid, her cancer comes back in other areas or stops responding to the treatments. We were again reminded that her cancer is a "chronic disease."

But we also heard him say he now thinks she can be one of the 10 percent that beats stage 4 cancer, and he stated strongly that his goal now is not just to control and manage her cancer but to beat it.

Second thing we heard was—and I'm not kidding—the sound of clapping. He showed us a graph of Susan's cancer markers and clapped his hands because he was so impressed with how Susan is responding to her treatments. Pure joy is how I would put his reaction.

In March Susan's markers were 432; as of July 16, they were at 89. Let me see if I can put this into perspective: her markers would have to climb 480 percent to get back to where they were just five months ago.

The reason for his excitement is the sharp and steady rate of the drop. He told us that this is not normal for someone with cancer as advanced as Susan's. Of course, Susan is having a hard time accepting this news.

Then we tried to talk about diet with him, but again he said, "Don't deprive yourself." I really like and respect Dr. Kashani, and I know he supports what we are doing; however, I am not sure he understands how much we have done and how important diet and other lifestyle changes can affect a cancer patient's outcome. All the changes we have made are backed by solid scientific evidence as to their effectiveness.

Many doctors are really good at what they do. They treat cancer with medicine and they know about most of the new drugs and treatments sitting on the horizon. However, most doctors have only forty-five hours of classroom study in nutrition, which is one class for one term. Consequently, I will continue to make that part of Susan's treatment my domain.

It makes me more determined to write the cookbook for cancer patients because I know that cancer patients are rarely counseled on what and how to eat. I know they likely won't be told to stop eating sugar, which is fuel for cancer cells, or processed foods, which are loaded with salt, sugar, artificial colorings and preservatives, and hydrogenated oils. And they certainly won't be given a list of foods that are known to fight cancer.

Snakes and Mangos
By Jeff Weaver — Sep 20, 2012, 3:05 p.m.
Susan sent me a text this morning letting me know she hurts. The aching in her joints is getting worse, her fingers hurt, and now the joints in her toes ache, too.

Even as the news gets better, the side effects of her chemo treatments team up with her cancer to remind us that this isn't over. Cancer is relentless.

It also reminds me that it is a one-day-at-a-time thing, and I need to stay focused on what I can do for Susan.

Just the other day Susan and I talked about her diet as I was peeling and cutting up a big, juicy mango. I joked with her that it was mango that made her better. And I added that if she ate papaya she would be better yet.

"Tastes like dirt," she said. It's nice that we can joke about this.

Well, not twenty minutes after getting her text, I came across a new study in which Texas researchers have found that extracts from peaches and plums killed breast cancer cells, even the most aggressive kinds, because of the amount of polyphenols in those fruits (Underground Health Reporter, September 20, 2012). Not only did the cancerous cells die but also none of the nearby healthy cells were affected.

Here is what they found: two specific phenols, chlorogenic and neochlorogenic, were responsible for this targeted killing of cancerous cells. Both are very common in fruits but more so in stone fruits such as plums, peaches, cherries, mangos, and papayas.

Then I came across an article on Fox News in the Health section about a joint British-Australian study on snake venom and gene sequencing (September 20, 2012). The researchers discovered that snake venom "evolved from regular cells but could be turned back into harmless proteins."

This discovery is important because snake venom uses "the same physiological pathways as human diseases." This opens up the possibilities for the development of new drugs for cancer and diabetes.

According to the study, certain snake venoms separate the cells that line blood vessels and kill them, "including the kinds that feed cancerous tumors." So, understanding how this works could lead to more effective cancer treatments.

I am constantly amazed at how all this stuff works and how these dedicated scientists continually find possible new ways to treat and hopefully cure cancer. And, more importantly, it fills me with hope that these studies will lead to cures for many who are fighting cancer.

I never thought I would ever say this in one sentence . . .

Thank God for rattlesnakes and mangos.

Racing for the Cure
By Jeff Weaver — Sep 24, 2012, 3:43 p.m.

Yesterday we took 7,111 steps. Give or take, depending on who was doing the walking.

More than thirty thousand good folks turned out at seven thirty in the morning on a bright sunny day in Newport Beach for the 5K Susan G. Komen Race for the Cure. People from all walks of life and all stages of cancer came. There were babies being pushed in strollers, preschoolers, grade schoolers, high schoolers, college kids, mothers and fathers, grandmothers and grandfathers, and I even saw one older gentleman in his seventies or eighties pushing his walker along with an oxygen bottle strapped to it and tubes in his nose.

They came to support the fight against cancer. They came to support loved ones with cancer and to celebrate those who have lost their battle with cancer.

But, as in life, not all was good. A few bitter, dare I say, ugly people came to protest the Susan G. Komen Foundation and to spew venom and hatred at everyone who passed them.

Nicki and Francesca came up with the idea to field a team for Susan. So, fifteen of us laced up our walking shoes, painted pink lines under our eyes, tied pink ribbons on our arms, pinned on race numbers and Susan Weaver signs, and took 7,111 steps in a show of support for Susan. To let her know she isn't traveling her road alone.

Let me see if I can capture some of the things and emotions I saw and felt. First, Fashion Island in Newport Beach is a great place to hold a fund-raising race.

Susan and I got there around six thirty and had to register and get our race numbers and signs. We each got white and pink t-shirts, and breast cancer survivors like Susan got a pink one. You are classified as a survivor the minute you are diagnosed with cancer, which seems kind of odd to me.

On our way to the starting line, it felt like we were a sports team going through the tunnel and out onto the field. The streets were lined with high school and college cheerleaders all decked out in their school's uniforms and doing cheers, waving pompoms. Dozens of regular folks had formed their own cheer squads and were dressed in homemade matching t-shirts cheering for the teams. People carried signs supporting various causes or individuals. The air was filled with the sounds of clapping and yelling and bands playing everything from rock to reggae. The announcer's voice boomed from loudspeakers, and big bunches of helium-filled balloons rose from the big arch across the starting line.

At the start of the race we counted down from ten to the gun. When the gun fired, there was genuine excitement and the mass of bodies surged forward like pink blood cells through an artery. As we headed down the first stretch, I was truly amazed at the number of people. For the most part, I walked behind our team and watched Susan as she walked beside her teammates. She went from one to another, talking, laughing, and putting her arm around them.

As we walked down the street, I was reminded how cruel and indiscriminate cancer is. Because the people fighting cancer and those who have fought it wore special pink t-shirts, I saw the many faces of cancer. Old women, young women, black, white, brown, and yellow women, and even a few men. They wore wigs, some had no hair at all, and some, like Susan, had supershort hair. They were tall or short, thin or overweight, and everywhere in between.

Not long after the start I saw Susan stop and talk to an elderly lady wearing her pink survivor shirt who seemed to be struggling to keep up. Susan reached out and took her hand and said something to her. I don't know what Susan said, but when she left, the lady had a big smile. As we headed up a hill, Kim Maffioli's young daughter Marina was getting hot and tired. Susan went over to her and gave her some encouragement and pointed out a little old man pushing his walker and oxygen bottle up the hill. She said, "If he can do it, so can we," and put her hand on Marina's shoulder and walked beside her.

I was worried about Susan. I wondered whether she had the strength to make it or if walking so far would sap the energy she needs to fight her cancer. But as I walked behind her I could see her *gain* strength from those around her. She was having a great time. She laughed and talked, joked around with Nicki, Sue, Kevin, and the other team members and with total strangers.

I saw a young mother pushing her three-year-old daughter in a stroller. A stream of bubbles came pouring out from under the stroller's blue hood. Some of the bubbles popped right away, some drifted down to the ground and sat there for an instant before popping, and some made their way through the mass of legs and arms and drifted up into the bright blue California sky. I watched as they drifted and turned, their translucent shells glistening and showing off their barely visible purple and blue and pink hues. I tried to take a picture of one, but I couldn't see it through my camera's viewfinder. It went so far up I lost sight of it.

And Now We Fight

As we neared the finish line, I saw dozens of signs hanging on palm trees and streetlight poles. Each sign had a picture and a short epitaph of someone who had lost the battle with cancer. Even though I was surrounded by celebration and laughter, I started to cry because every picture was of a smiling face, and every message was one of honor. I looked around and saw hundreds of men and women wearing pink survivor t-shirts, and I prayed that their pictures would never be up there. I said a little extra prayer asking that Susan's would never be there either. And then I watched Susan walk alongside Nicki. My two favorite girls side by side, both deeply invested in this very personal fight. I had to step away from the throng of marchers for a few seconds. And, yes, I smudged the pink face paint under my eyes. For the life of me, I can't understand why I have such a hard time containing my emotions.

At the end of the race, we approached the big balloon archway that was the finish line. Hundreds of people were there to greet and high-five us. About twenty feet before we crossed the line, I walked up to Susan and lifted her up into my arms and carried her across the line. Not because she was tired, which she was, but because I wanted her to know that no matter what it takes I will be there for her and together we will finish life's race on our terms, not cancer's.

Later, I asked Susan what she thought of the whole thing. She wanted to thank everyone who spent their hard-earned money to support and honor her and to support the fight against cancer. Thanks to Nicki and Kevin, Francesca and Ryan, Francesca's sister-in-law, Lisa, who is pregnant and due today! And Sue, Michelle and Jeremiah, Amy and Melissa, Natalie, Kim and her daughter, Marina. I hope I didn't forget anyone.

She also said this: "It made me tired! Seriously, once again I am astounded because of everyone's support and friendship and how much they care and are willing to sacrifice and give for me. That was a lot both physically and monetarily (forty dollars for each entrant). I wish there was a way for every penny to go to research and to education about diet. And I want to address the protesters at the end of the race. They said there's no hope and no cure—that pissed me off! And that it's been seventy-five years with no cure—that's flat out wrong. Cancer is curable with early detection because of new medicine. Plus, there have been tremendous advances and more all the time. If we give up, then there will never be a cure. Twenty years ago there would have been nothing they could have done for me. And they didn't know just how important diet was. So, all the money being given to charities, like the Susan G. Komen Foundation, *is* helping. We can't just quit because there isn't a cure for all types of cancer yet. Don't give up!"

Yesterday, we all took steps to help find a cure, to help those cancer patients in need pay bills and buy food, and to put one foot in front of the other in the fight against cancer . . . 7,111 steps each.

For some reason I can't stop thinking of that one bubble, the one that floated high into the sky. If only there was a way to make their shells stronger so more of them would be with us much longer . . . as they make their way toward heaven.

Learning to Live with Cancer: The Next Step Forward
By Jeff Weaver — Oct 5, 2012, 4:15 p.m.

The road to normalcy continues. Susan is getting a little stronger each week. Of course, she still has bad days mixed in with the good ones, but thankfully the good ones now outnumber the bad.

Monday she will be returning to work. Both of us are excited that she has progressed far enough for that to happen. This is a major hallmark for her. She is returning to a more "normal" routine. And that is what we have prayed for all along . . . to be normal again.

However, both Susan and I now have a new and real concern. How will she hold up under the daily stresses of her job? First, there is the physical stress because the job involves a lot of hard work, and even when she was "normal" she got tired. Susan is prone to giving everything she has, and she pushes herself every day. It is one of the reasons why she is so good at what she does.

Then, there is the mental part of the work. That will tax her even more. I'm sure she is going to try to overcompensate for her absence. Last, the hours. Not so much the number of hours she works, but how early she must get up. She needs to be up and running before five in the morning, and that really worries me because she won't get enough sleep. She still has the hot flash thing going on. Because she is on estrogen therapy, she gets superhot all through the night, making sleep very difficult.

It's important that Susan is well rested. She needs all her strength to continue her fight. Even though the news has been great lately, we cannot forget she is still a stage 4 cancer patient and that her cancer can still put up a fight. This stuff does not go away quietly, if at all. Studies show that stress and fatigue are detrimental to a cancer patient's recovery.

Something we will do now is to make sure she eats foods that will give her more energy. That means more proteins early in the morning and complex carbohydrates throughout the day so her blood sugar level doesn't drop. We will prepare as much as we can the night before so she can stay in bed longer. I will need to kick her out of the kitchen again so she can rest when she gets home from work. It's been nice for me lately because for a few weeks now she has been strong enough to do the cooking.

And the toughest thing is I will need to convince her to cut her hair. Yes, it's getting too long. Short hair means she can sleep ten or fifteen minutes longer.

She will still be receiving her treatments for the foreseeable future, so that means one to two weeks of aching bones, joints that hurt, fatigue, and of course the hot flashes. Going forward, we will be keeping a very close watch on her cancer markers. If they spike up, we'll have to make adjustments.

We are entering new territory here. We hope everything goes smoothly and without any setbacks. One of my biggest worries is that all the added stress and fatigue could open the door for her cancer and how that would affect her mind-set if it were to come back. She has fought so hard to get to this point.

We are only in the third round of this heavyweight fight.

Now this is for Susan: I love how you look with your hair short. Would you please get it cut? Just for me, okay?

One More Step, Back at Work
By Jeff Weaver — Oct 17, 2012, 3:43 p.m.

It's been a full week since Susan went back to work. In my opinion it's a good news, bad news sorta thing. First, let me get the bad out of the way. *Bad* may be overstating it a little. I worry that Susan will get run down and that will reduce her body's ability to fight off the cancer cells that we know are lurking inside her. Even after just one week I can see the effects getting up so early and eight hours of physical exertion have had on her.

Now, the good news. Susan has purpose, something to help take her mind off her disease. She was again reminded of how much people care and how much support she has. When she got home from work after her first day, she was full of energy and there was a big smile on her face. I asked her if she was tired, and she said no, she didn't get to work much because she was too busy getting hugs and giving updates to her coworkers.

After dinner, rather than resting, she started to go through two big, three-ring binders. I asked what they were. She said, "Oh, just stuff for work." She was going over all the old and new merchandise. She wanted to know what had changed in her absence. Now, how many people take stuff home with them so they can do a better job? But that's my Susan.

On Tuesday, her second day back, she had to take the day off. She had an issue that required a visit to the doctor. Thankfully, it was nothing serious. But here's the deal: that something serious can happen at any moment is always a possibility. Every little lump or new pain has to be watched closely.

Even though Susan's life is returning to an old familiar routine, she will never really feel normal again. Uncertainty and constant fear are part of living with cancer.

Bonfires, Cancer, and Reality
By Jeff Weaver — Oct 25, 2012, 5:28 p.m.

Tomorrow Susan, Nicki, Josh, and I are going to Oregon for a family reunion. Back when the kids were small my dad had a big bonfire every October. He would pile all the old brush and boards up in the bottom pasture, and it was always a big pile. Just before dark everyone would gather around and eagerly await the moment when Dad would ignite the twenty-foot-high pile. We all felt the excitement, especially the youngest children. But truth be told, I think some of us older folks were even more excited. I remember the flames going up twenty to thirty feet high.

Dad always parked the old wooden hay trailer nearby, and on it were ice chests full of sodas (maybe even a cold beer or two) and sacks of chips, hot dogs, and of course marshmallows. He had dozens of long sharpened sticks next to the hot dogs. After the fire burned down to a big heap of hot, glowing red coals, the kids would grab the sticks and start roasting the treats.

Dad would fuss over the kids and the fire. Every time he would stir the coals, the embers would rise high into the dark night sky, leaving shimmering red trails.

This will be the last bonfire. Dad is eighty-six and slowing down. Because Mom's health and memory aren't the best and with Susan's cancer, he wanted all of us together before . . . well, before it's too late.

I came across a new study this morning that was sobering. It had an unexpected impact on me. I have been so confident about Susan's recovery. It's as if I have forgotten about where she was just seven months ago when her doctor softly told her, "We can't cure you, only extend your life."

I'm not sure why I am writing this. Maybe it's to give us all a reality check and to point out again just how important it is to do everything in your power to PREVENT cancer rather than try to cure it.

I read an article on Reuters that dealt with how a majority of people with incurable cancer think that their chemotherapy treatments will cure their cancer (June 5, 2012).

In some cases the treatments are designed only to extend their lives. The study, reported in the *New England Journal of Medicine*, found that a majority of the patients' expectations were far too high. Patients who were terminal didn't know that the chemotherapy would not kill their tumors. Sadly, the treatments will only give the patients a very short amount of time that's filled with terrible side effects.

Part of the study deals with how doctors communicate with their patients. (I, for one, can tell you it is a complex dynamic because I've been through this twice now.) It's hard for doctors to tell a patient they can't cure the cancer. Often, when doctors fully inform their patients, most patients don't believe what they are told. But, what is worse, some doctors don't inform their patients that their cancer is incurable or they don't make it clear how dire the situation is.

It was also found that when people are diagnosed with incurable cancer many of them think they are going to beat the odds.

And when I read that, it made we wonder whether Susan and I are just kidding ourselves by being too optimistic.

Dr. Asuncion had told us what the deal was, and she was kind when she delivered the news. But we chose to be optimistic, we refused to take that news lying down, and we have been proactive in our fight against Susan's cancer.

I mean, what are we supposed to do? Accept the death sentence and wait around to die? One thing I do know, we are going to fight harder. I wish we would have made changes to our diet years ago, and then maybe Susan wouldn't have to have drugs pumped into her that do more harm than good and that statistically have been shown not to be able to cure her.

We also are going to live every single day knowing that there is a chance Susan will beat her cancer.

With this in mind, Susan and I are looking forward to visiting family and friends and standing out in the field by the bonfire.

Here is what we won't be doing: eating any hotdogs or sugary marshmallows or drinking sugary sodas. And we won't be telling others what they should or shouldn't eat, at least not this weekend.

As for me, this study is a harsh reminder that Susan is dealing with a deadly serious condition. You can bet your life that I will enjoy every single glowing ember that floats up into the night sky this Saturday night. I'll hold Susan tight so I can feel her warmth, and I'll tell her I love her. Hell, I might even give the old man a big hug to boot.

Hot Time Down on the Farm
By Jeff Weaver — Nov 1, 2012, 5:14 p.m.
Well, we made it home. But what a trip it was. The bonfire was exactly like I remember it. I am not sure how many showed up, but I'll take a guess, fifty or more.

It's a fourteen-hour-plus trip from Orange County to Myrtle Creek. We got in Friday evening and checked into the Seven Feather's Hotel and Casino. I have to say, the hotel is very nice.

Our diet makes it very hard to travel and still eat like we need to. But Jennifer, my sister, told us to go to the Creek Side Restaurant, where she is a chef, which is part of the Seven Feathers complex. They had some good vegan dishes.

Saturday morning I got up early and took a four-mile walk out Gazley Road, which runs along the South Umpqua River. It was dark and raining, so I got soaked. I forgot how nice clean, fresh air is. As I walked past a couple of the farms, I came to an apple tree that was loaded with fruit. When I was in high school, we would stop at that tree and run out into the farmer's yard and pick a few apples. The apples were tasty, but it was the "danger" of swiping the fruit that made us do it. Well, I couldn't resist the temptation to relive my wild youth, so I looked around to make sure no one would see me and snuck over to the apple tree and grabbed a couple. Guess what? It's still kind of exciting and the apples I swiped were delicious. Oh, and it's a good thing I've lost lots of weight; otherwise, I might not have outrun the farmer's dog that wanted to take a bite out of my recently downsized ass.

After my walk Susan and I visited with a few of my old friends, Tim and Patty Kelley and Nick and Linda Counts. Then we went over to Dad's place.

That afternoon, cousins, nieces and nephews, and their families started showing up. It wasn't long before Dad had a full house. A couple hours before dark he went down to the lower field where he had the wood piled for the fires and started a small cooking fire. Soon the rest of us went down.

I was surprised at all the little ones. Because I'm not around, I've lost track of just how big our family is. My oldest son, Curtis, and his wife, Siony, and their baby, Cody, came down from Eagle Point. It was the first time I've seen Cody (he is eighteen months now), other than in photos. He is nearly as big as his mom.

The best part for me was seeing everyone interact with Susan. She was getting hugs and lots of encouragement. And I can't tell you how many times I heard "You look great." Her short hair seems to be a big hit.

It was also bittersweet because I think everyone knew this may be the last time they saw Mom. She is not doing well and it shows because she looks really frail. But Mom had a great time, and every single person there spent a good deal of time with her. She looked like and acted like she knew us all. But I know she didn't and that was heartbreaking.

I took some time to sit with her and talk. She still has her sense of humor and enjoys recounting embarrassing things from our childhood.

Just as I remembered, Dad had the old Farmall tractor with its steel seat worn to a shine by four generations of jeans and the wooden hay trailer out there. On the trailer were boxes of sodas and hotdogs and marshmallows and sharpened roasting sticks. It wasn't long before hotdogs were roasting over the red hot coals. Then the kids started making s'mores. Everyone was respectful of Susan's diet, so that was good.

Just before dark Dad lit the bonfire. The flames must have reached thirty or forty feet high. We could feel the heat from way, way back. But the fire wasn't the only source of warmth. Like every family, we have our issues now and again, but not that night. It was terrific. Everyone was telling stories, laughing, and we all caught up on each other's lives.

More importantly, Susan had a great time and she again found out how much she is loved.

We stayed until the fire burned down. After the flames died down enough, we all pulled up lawn chairs around the huge pile of glowing red and blue and white hot coals. It was close to midnight before we left.

On Sunday, Cammy Davis, one of Susan's old friends, and her mom, Carol, drove down from Jacksonville. They had a long visit. Later in the day Susan drove up to Yoncalla to visit with Kimberly Robins, another old friend. Kim wanted Susan to go horseback riding, but time was running short.

When she got back to Dad's place, we all sat around talking for a couple hours. Time seemed to fly by, and before I knew it, it was time to get back to the hotel because we were planning on leaving early, like four a.m. early.

As we said our goodbyes, Dad gave Susan a hug. He looked down at her and said, "You take care of yourself, sis." I could tell he had to hold back tears, and so did Susan. And for anyone who knows my dad, that's something.

Cancer Risk and Breast Density
By Jeff Weaver — Nov 18, 2012, 11:54 p.m.

Last night I was thinking about all the studies I've read on the things that increase the risk of cancer in humans. I wondered whether we missed a key warning sign that Susan may have been more at risk than others. Was it her diet, where we lived, or environmental factors? Or was she just unlucky? Or could it have been that she has dense breasts? The fact that she has had lumps before made me wonder whether there was some correlation between dense breasts and cancer risk. So, I did a little digging.

It turns out there is a connection between breast cancer risk and breast density. I came across a 2007 study on this published in the *New England Journal of Medicine*.

The study found that women with dense breasts, which means there is a lot more fibrous or glandular tissue and not enough fat in the breast, were five times more likely to contract breast cancer than were women with less-dense breasts. That is a very significant difference. The report went so far as to say that "women are being left dangerously in the dark about a cancer risk" and that it was "the best kept secret." In fact, the study found that only 5 percent of women know they have dense breasts, and only nineteen states require doctors to tell women they do and the risk associated with it.

Well, that set off alarm bells. Susan has dense breasts, and she had lumps long before she was diagnosed with cancer; however, we never heard from her doctor that she was at a greater risk because of this. In fact, we were told not to worry.

It certainly seems to me that it would be prudent to inform all women about their breast density and the accompanying risk factor, especially if it is discovered by a routine mammogram.

I am sure if Susan and I had been told about this risk we would have kept a closer eye on any changes, done more self-examinations, and paid an extra visit to the doctor every so often.

It would be wise for all women to find out whether they have dense breasts and then act accordingly.

Thanksgiving Potpourri
By Jeff Weaver — Nov 22, 2012, 3:03 p.m.
So, here we are, nearly nine months to the day since Susan was diagnosed with cancer. It changed our lives forever and the lives of many others.

It's Thanksgiving already. On one hand, it seems like this year has gone by so fast yet at the same time not fast enough. What I mean is, with everything that has happened to our family this year, it feels like we haven't had time to breathe between doctor appointments, chemo sessions, surgeries, and the other out-of-the-ordinary things we have done or participated in, such as Susan's fund-raisers, cancer walks, visits from Ann, and our trip to Oregon. It's been a blur of activities. On the other hand, I find myself praying that all this would be over, that we could go back to being just a regular family with normal problems. I keep thinking about the five-year mark: if a cancer patient makes it that long, her odds of surviving increase. If only Susan can get to her five-year anniversary and be cancer free.

And that makes me stop and think. I'm wishing her life away, in a sense, because, what if things take a turn for the worse?

I've been thinking a lot about this conundrum, and it dawned on me that this may have been one of the *best* years of our lives. We have learned so much about who we are as people and as a family. We've been blessed beyond anything I could have ever imagined. So, I thought I would ask a few people how Susan's cancer battle has affected them. I asked a couple of Susan's coworkers about the changes they made in diet.

Ryan and Francesca stayed at our home and looked after Mick and Jessie while we were in Oregon. This is from Ryan:

Francesca had mentioned that you wanted something for the journal about our lifestyle changes. Eating a vegan diet is something that we had never really considered. The word vegan *to us used to sound like "political activist" rather than "healthy lifestyle." We always wondered how someone could have such an extreme diet. However, after reading the cookbook* Forks Over Knives *that was left out on your kitchen table, I was convinced. It seemed easy enough: eat foods that are plant based. It seemed like a no-brainer, and I asked Francesca, "Why haven't we been eating like this for years?" The recipes look great, and I'm sure the benefits far outweigh anything that we're currently eating. I now catch myself reading labels at the grocery store.*

Franny made spaghetti squash on Sunday. It was delicious, but it would have been better with Susan's homemade sauce. Nevertheless, my family loved it, and they were curious about our new health kick. Who would have thought that Susan's lifestyle change could positively affect so many others? Thanks, Susan and Jeff.

From Diane Olsen:

I got some good news recently when I visited my doctor. Along with the usual blood pressure and other vital checks, I was happy when I found out that my cholesterol has become somewhat lower. I'm pleased to know that the diet changes I've made are working.

I've been eating kale, beans, nongluten carbs, a lot of fiber, wheat pasta, and I don't remember the last time I had regular milk. When I do need milk for something, I go for the almond milk now and I'm getting used to it and I like it. It took a little while to make the changes a habit, but they are now, so I don't even have to think about it anymore. I highly recommend making these changes to lower your cholesterol!

Last night I talked on the phone to Penny Douglas, and she told me about her changes. Penny is a breast cancer survivor. She just had her five-year anniversary and checkup. She is still clear. Here is the gist of our conversation.

When I asked about her diet changes, she told me that she makes a smoothie everyday with lots of healthy greens and fruit in it. It sounded good. She has high blood pressure and cholesterol levels, so she hopes that by changing her eating habits that will help. She said she is a lot more conscious of what she eats and that she wants to make even more changes in her diet. She also said it was hard for her because she is the only one in her house that is doing this. Then our conversation turned to Susan and what it's like to find out you have cancer.

One thing she said was that when she was diagnosed no one told her anything about what to eat and what not to eat. Now she finds that incredulous. She told me how shocked she was when she found out about her cancer, because she thought she lived a good lifestyle with plenty of exercise and she thought she ate pretty well. She told me how afraid she was and how she still worries, even after five years with no recurrence.

Then she told me how much she admires Susan's strength. She is amazed at how hard Susan works even after all she has gone through and how dedicated she is to her eating habits. Then she brought up how amazing and radiant Susan looks, it's like she never had cancer at all. She said Susan is a real inspiration to everyone at Macy's and that everyone was praying for and pulling for her.

Last week I talked to my dear friends, Patty and Tim Kelley. Patty had a hip replacement on November 1, and Tim had a hernia operation on the fifteenth. I asked how they were doing, and they said great. Then Patty told me about a friend who was diagnosed with stage 3 breast cancer earlier this year. Patty said her friend went on a plant-based, whole foods diet. Just two weeks ago she was told she is 100 percent cancer free now!

Now a word from The Boss, Susan.

Thanksgiving. I love it. The food, the cooler weather, all the family around. But this year is a lot different. I don't get to bake pies and big dinner rolls and there will be no turkey that makes my dogs drool. Bummer. So, why am I still happy it's here? Because I'm still here, and I wasn't too sure I would be or, if I was, would be feeling very good. I can't even begin to tell all of you how thankful I am for what you have done for me. The prayers, the moral support, calling me and texting me, all the cards. It's amazing how much even the little things helped me mentally. Then there is the financial support. Wow! I would never have thought you could help so much. I don't know how I could have made it without you. I truly believe you have saved my life. I could not have paid for all my medical care without you. So, on Thanksgiving I am thankful for my life, my friends, my coworkers, my family and my in-laws, my kids, and my husband. And I'm thankful I've learned how blessed I am to have all of you in my life. Somehow during my life I have managed to surround myself with the most incredible people in the world. I don't deserve you, but I've got you, you're mine, and I will never give you up. I love you so much. Thanks for loving me, too.

Finally, I wanted to finish this entry by going back to something I said earlier: why this may be the best year of our lives despite Susan's battle with cancer. This year we learned a lot about our friends and family when things got rough.

I've learned I have the best in-laws. Ann and Marty are wonderful people, and they are loving and caring parents. I've always told everyone how lucky I am to have them as in-laws. I have a great family as well, from my mom and dad to all my brothers and sisters and the nieces and nephews and cousins. It's a really big family, and I love them all.

I have learned that Susan has incredible friends. Susan is right, we would have never made it without them, so thanks to you all.

I learned that my children are truly special. Of course, I always knew that, but, man, I have to say just how proud I am of them. They stepped up and pitched in and took on more than anyone their ages should have had to shoulder. Susan always worried that she wasn't the best mom, that she didn't do enough for them as they grew up. Well, the proof, as they say, is in the pudding. Josh and Nicole, you two are more than any parent could hope for.

But I think what I found out this year is just who I married. I learned how incredibly strong Susan is and how vulnerable as well. I learned how determined she can be, yet she still needed a little push now and again. I saw her courage in the darkest of hours and witnessed her deepest fears. I saw how compassionate she can be, how she is willing to put others' needs in front of hers, I saw her love of family and friends. I saw a power in her that I've never seen before. I saw a different kind of beauty in her, one that comes from the inside, and anyone who looks close enough can see it. I don't think she has ever looked more beautiful. And I saw her come of age and grow as someone truly worthy of admiration and respect. Best of all, I saw her and I grow even closer together. It has made me realize that without her, I would be lost and empty.

So, on this Thanksgiving Day I am thankful for my family and friends and I'm thankful that Susan kept me around all these years. And I promise to do everything in my power to make sure she is here for years to come.

51 and Counting
By Jeff Weaver — Dec 1, 2012, 8:19 a.m.
51. Ain't it a beautiful thing? I know that sounds silly, it's just a number, right? But for Susan it's an important number.

Yesterday we saw Susan's oncologist, Dr. Kashani. He came bouncing into the room, apologized several times for being late, and then he couldn't contain his excitement. He said, "I want to congratulate both of you, you are doing such a great job. . . . Look,

I want to show you something." Then he opened Susan's file and pulled up her last blood work. He pointed to her marker test and put it in a graph for us.

"See, right here, see how beautiful this is. I'm so impressed with the job you've done. Your CA 27-29 cancer markers have come from 432 all the way down to 51 . . . it's unbelievable how well you are responding to your treatments."

I looked at Susan and we both breathed a big sigh of relief. Funny thing is we weren't as excited as he was at first.

On the way down, I was so afraid of what we might hear this time. Susan has been worrying about a cough she has and the pain in her bones and joints but especially about her weight loss, or her perceived weight loss. (She's been between 108 and 104 for months.) Everyone keeps telling her she's so skinny. Now to most of us that might sound good, but for Susan it sets off alarm bells because weight loss could be a sign that her cancer may be back. This is one example of not realizing the effects your words have, especially when talking to a cancer patient.

You might think after all the good news we've had the last couple visits I wouldn't be so worried. However, Susan can't help but worry, and she's a bit of a skeptic. Her psyche is pretty darn fragile now, too. I have to keep her in a positive state of mind. It's a big deal. Science has proven that people who remain positive have better health and they recover better than those who have a negative attitude.

This fight is as much mental as it is physical or medical. I know that truly believing in what you are doing results in a higher degree of success. I worry that if I were to have a recurrence, she would lose faith in the plan we have been following. After all, I have made all the same lifestyle changes she has, so in her mind it would mean that these changes won't work for her either.

All that said, we are happy that her cancer markers are down. Susan asked Dr. Kashani what "normal" was. He told her that 39 was normal for the breast cancer marker CA 27-29. Let's see: in March her markers were 432, in April, 230, in July, 91, in September, 71, and on November 5, they were down to 51. From last July to the present, every three months there has been a twenty-point drop. Hmm, so at this rate 39 is just around the corner.

She is inching her way toward being in remission. We will remain steadfast in our efforts. Last night she told me that if she could have anything at all, it would be to be normal again: like she was before cancer. Well, I know she will never be like she was before, but . . .

Twelve more points down, baby. That is normal, and that makes 12 even more beautiful than

51!

Time Keeps on Slippin' Away
By Jeff Weaver — Dec 31, 2012, 5:26 p.m.

Every year around this time, it seems as if people are compelled to remark on the passage of time. "I can't believe it's December already!" or "How is the year almost over?" are common statements in the weeks and months leading up to the new calendar year.

This year, amid all the talk of debt bubbles, elections, and fiscal cliffs, I suspect that some folks wish time would move a little faster so we could get past these weighty issues. However, for most of us, we try to ignore that stuff.

In that lies danger. Because when we let our guard down, time is free to make fools of us. So, any opportunity for sincere reflection, no matter the impetus, is something I think everyone should take time for.

Looking back, I can kick myself for not reading the signals Susan was sending. She started saying things like "It doesn't matter because I probably won't be around to . . ." She kept telling me that Jessie (our red Aussie) was clinging to her and smelling her. She became unusually pessimistic about everything. I think a blind man could have seen she was trying to tell me something was wrong. Now I am becoming a much better listener and I try to watch body language.

Time has a way of sorting out the wheat from the chaff. There are so many images I have of Susan, but some have really stuck with me. Like the night I sat and watched her lie on the couch with a blanket pulled up to her head, sick and shaking. Or the night I came to bed and she was lying balled up in a fetal position, bald head resting uncomfortably on her pillow, hurting right down to the deepest part of her bones. I couldn't help feeling like our time was coming to an end. But she never gave up.

Even with those kinds of images burned into my brain—and there are hundreds of them—I think some others, better ones, are even more lasting. I really love the picture I took of Susan whispering in Josh's ear after her first chemo treatment. And the day I sat and watched her standing at the window looking at the baby birds in their nest in the hanging flowerpot. She was talking so softly and lovingly to them. As I watched her, I knew I had a very special woman for a wife and one who had been forever changed.

Time flew by. Treatments and more treatments, and infections, and surgeries and doctor appointments. It felt like we lived at Sand Canyon Medical Center. Ann came and went, but what a visit it was, and she made the most traumatic time for all of us more bearable. I can only imagine what it must have been like for Ann. But time moves relentlessly on and so did we.

Each visit to the doctor was one of hope and worry. We worried that the news would be bad but hoped it would continue to be better than the last visit's. And it was. Susan's numbers kept getting better and better. Around September we allowed ourselves to start thinking seriously about Susan beating her cancer. Still, the odds were against her, but we thought all the treatments she has had and the expertise of her doctors, along with all Susan has done in the way of diet and exercise, plus her astounding willpower, and with God's graces, might buy us time.

And that leads me to this. . . .

This year is done. Its time has slipped away and we are left only with its memories. I will never be able to forget some things, and some things I never want to forget.

I will never take Susan's time here for granted or, for that matter,

Josh's and Nicole's. It feels almost like a great weight has been lifted from us. We all know this is not over yet, but I think we may have been given a second chance.

So, tonight as we sit home, watching the clock tick away, Susan and I will have a long talk about what was and what will be. And I am going to promise her these things:

A better year. As much love as I can muster. And that I will savor every last second with her, even if it is just watching the time slip into the past while dreaming of our future.

Time is a precious commodity. And we only have so much of it allotted to us. I am thankful mine will be spent alongside Susan. Like she told me once, "We are a pretty good team."

Amen, baby!

Learning to Live with Cancer: New Mortality Study
By Jeff Weaver — Jan 8, 2013, 4:40 p.m.

Yesterday I read a new study, and parts of it concerned me a little. Last night Susan and I had a talk about what we have done, where we needed to be more vigilant, and what our goals were going forward—a sort of strategy session, if you will.

I thought I would highlight parts of the study here. And share a few of our thoughts and concerns.

The United States is in the fiftieth year of its "war on cancer," and deaths from cancer continue to decline.

At first glance, the findings in the report, published in the *Journal of the National Cancer Institute*, seem very encouraging.

However, experts from the National Cancer Institute, the American Cancer Society, and other groups say the report doesn't tell the whole story on the progress. They believe that the decline in death rates is due to the sharp decline in smoking rather than the billions of dollars spent to discover and implement advanced cancer treatments.

The report pointed out that bad diets, lack of physical activity, and obesity are the reasons mortality rates aren't going down faster. The researchers believed that these lifestyle choices and conditions will supplant smoking as the leading causes of cancer in the United States in the decades ahead.

Many experts think we haven't made much progress, considering the billions of dollars spent on finding a cure for cancer, along with all the information the public now can access, when compared to the minimally small annual reductions in cancer death rates.

The percentage of deaths from all types of cancer has been declining since the early 1990s, by about 1.8 percent per year in men and 1.4 percent per year in women. But progress has stalled even as expensive new drugs and potential new treatment methods have been introduced. The death rates for men from 2005 to 2009 was unchanged at 1.8 percent, and for women, a slightly higher 1.5 percent.

The question is why?

Now I am no expert on this, but everything I have read indicates the typical lifestyles of Americans have changed, specifically diet, to the point that people diagnosed with cancer counteract their treatments by eating and drinking foods that in essence create a Petrie dish for cancer proliferation.

It is reasonable to conclude that the number of people who will be diagnosed with cancer will increase in the coming decades. We are under more stress today than ever before, we consume ten times more sugar than just twenty years ago, fast food has become a large part of our daily diets, we eat more processed foods and far less natural and healthy foods, and there is a huge increase in people who are obese. Plus, we have become more sedentary. All these are contributing factors for cancer.

What worries me the most is, as the study points out, cancer's unique ability, even as it is being decimated by one drug, to learn and then circumvent the treatment and find new ways to thrive, proliferate, and attack with greater potency than at first. When I thought about everything Susan is up against, I started to have some doubts. And I asked myself, are we fooling ourselves? Are we doing everything possible to give her the best chance? And if her cancer comes back, what then?

Last Friday I took Susan to her treatment. She had all three of them this time, the three-hour Aredia drip and the Lupron and Faslodex shots. Sitting there beside her as she goes through her personal hell is a stark reminder that this is no joke; this is still a life-and-death struggle. One she will fight for the foreseeable future.

Because, as the study points out, cancer learns and adapts and then continues to elude everything some of the best minds in the world with billions of dollars throw at it. It is an insidious disease that is relentless and deadly.

If we really want to decrease Susan's odds of dying from cancer, then we need to strictly adhere to the major changes in lifestyle we made.

One thing that is abundantly clear to me after reading all these studies is this: the biggest reductions in cancer mortality will come from prevention rather than treatment.

Just some food for thought as we continue learning how to live with cancer.

Happy Birthday, Baby!
By Jeff Weaver — Jan 22, 2013, 1:23 p.m.
Today is Susan's birthday. She turns forty-nine. I can see some of you cringe because I just wrote down her age and I know how some people (you girls!) don't like acknowledging your age. But this time I'm willing to take the butt chewing that is probably coming.

Birthdays were never a big deal when I was growing up. I don't recall ever having a birthday party or one for my brothers and sisters. But when I met Susan, that changed because after the birth of our son, Josh, we have always celebrated birthdays.

This morning I looked at some old photos of birthdays over the years. One was of Susan lying in a hospital bed holding Josh the day he was born, with his tiny foot resting in her hand. There were chocolate cakes. Josh and Nicole blowing out candles. Huge smiles and faces covered with chocolate frosting. Bright and colorful balloons. I saw pure joy.

Susan made sure we celebrated. She made birthdays special days at our house. They were days we looked forward to.

What I didn't see were any pictures of Susan's birthdays—not because we didn't celebrate them but because she always downplayed her own birthday.

Seeing all those old photos of Susan and the kids made me wonder what Ann and Marty were thinking today. I am sure they have special memories of days long past, of cakes and balloons and presents and joy. Maybe at this moment Ann is sitting looking at a picture of Susan with chocolate cake all over her face. I think our children's birthdays are somehow more important to us than our own.

Susan is alive and may be gaining the upper hand in her fight, and that makes today special. But I am torn as to what I should do. Should I go all out or do what we always do? If I go all out, will she think I am worried that she may not have any more birthdays? Will she fret that she is forty-nine or be thankful she made it to forty-nine? (I'm guessing both.)

I have a few hours to decide what to do before she gets home from work. I do know this: I'll try to find the perfect card, I'll get her a small gift, and maybe I'll bake her some sugar-free cookies made with something other than refined flour and eggs.

And there is one more thing I am going to do. I'm going to take a few minutes and pray to God to ask him if he would make sure to keep her around for many more years. Because without her, birthdays just won't be the same.

Happy birthday, baby. I love you.

Birds and Cookies and Soup
By Jeff Weaver — Jan 25, 2013, 4:48 p.m.
Every morning I feed my birds. I put some wild bird food out on the table on the back patio and then go inside, sit down, and drink my coffee as I watch the birds flock in and eat. Then, without any reason that I can see, they all vanish in a heartbeat. Seeds and chaff scatter all over. They are a jumpy lot! They startle over the

smallest things, things I can't hear or see.

Yesterday morning I went out to move my plant seedlings (I'm growing chard and kale) to catch the morning sun when I noticed a huge red-tailed hawk sitting in the top of a big pine tree on the slope right behind the house. He was peering down at my birds. He was waiting for them to slip up, waiting for that one opportunity to strike should they let their guard down.

I went back in to get another cup of coffee, and I saw the cookies I had baked for Susan's birthday sitting on the counter. She loved them! I had taken a couple recipes and started substituting healthy ingredients. I ended up with cookies that had no sugar, butter, eggs, or white flour, and I used sugar-free dark chocolate with 85 percent cacao.

Looking at those cookies made me think about something Drew Hilliard, the young Navy lieutenant, posted on his blog about his fight with cancer. Last week he wrote that some suspicious-looking spots showed up on his last scan. He has been clear for two years; however, he and his doctors are worried the spots may be trouble.

One thing he wrote that really got my attention was that he was going to stop eating sugar . . . again. Apparently, he let his guard down as far as diet goes. So, now he's going to watch his diet again. It's the *again* that got my attention.

I worry about whether I am being picky enough with Susan. I want her to have a wide variety of foods, and I want her to have some of the things she loves, like honey and bread and cake and chocolate chip cookies.

There is the temptation sometimes to say, well, just this one time won't hurt or to throw together something quick and easy when I am short on time or tired. But here's the deal. Is it really worth it to tempt fate like that? It is sort of like thumbing our noses at cancer.

That is a dangerous game. Cancer has a mind of its own and it can reinvent itself to get around any treatment. It's like Arnold in *The Terminator*. You can knock him down but can't kill him.

So, why on earth would we play such a dangerous game with what we eat? This is serious business, and we can't let our guard down for one minute. The point is, it is wise to be like my birds and to be overly cautious. They know it's better to keep an eye on the hawk and take preventative actions before they find themselves in a battle that they most likely won't win.

Immortality and the Food You Choose
By Jeff Weaver — Jan 31, 2013, 2:01 p.m.
"Immortality is the sole domain of the Gods."

That is how Patrick Cox opened a piece titled "Virtual Immortality" in his newsletter, the *Penny Sleuth* (January 30, 2013).

But we all have thought about what it would be like to be immortal. To live forever.

Sorry to say, that's the stuff of fanciful dreams, reserved for those warm nights lying under a sky filled with millions of stars. Times when you can afford to let your mind wander the universe, dreaming of god-like things.

However, as we know, we all can do certain things that increase the odds of us living longer and in better health. I just read an article on Fox News in the Health section titled "Vegetarians Slash Risk of Heart Disease." (January 31, 2013). It discussed a new study on diet and how everyone can prolong their lives by eliminating the risk of heart disease and cancer by what they choose to eat.

Researchers at the University of Oxford found that vegetarians are much less likely to suffer from serious heart disease than people who eat meat, including fish. They analyzed forty-five thousand volunteers from the 1990s until 2009. The study found that the risk of heart disease in vegetarians is about 32 percent lower than in people who eat meat and fish.

The article points out that "the study took into account factors such as age, smoking, alcohol intake, physical activity, educational level and socioeconomic background, and recorded the blood pressure and cholesterol levels of participants."

The researchers concluded that "overwhelmingly, vegetarians had lower blood pressure, cholesterol levels, and body mass indexes than non-vegetarians."

In another study conducted in Brisbane, Australia, researchers found that a diet of mainly leafy greens, dark-colored fruits and vegetables, along with whole grains and legumes reduced the risk of cancer by 75 percent and in some cases aided in the reversal of certain types of cancer.

The study had twenty-five hundred noncancerous volunteers, half of whom maintained a traditional diet and the other half of whom ate mainly a whole foods, plant-based diet. They also studied advanced-stage cancer patients.

In the group with advanced cancer, half of the 450 patients were on the normal Western diet and half converted to a plant-based diet. The researchers found that in the plant-based group death rates were 15 percent less after ten years, life spans were extended for 42 percent of the volunteers, and they had fewer side effects from treatments.

The results of these studies mirror hundreds of other studies. I think we can say that the science on diet in relation to heart disease and cancer is settled.

Eating a plant-based diet buys time for most all of us. But immortality? That's different. A pipe dream, most would say.

Well, maybe not. Researchers are now working on a therapy that could reverse the age of individual cells by using stem cells that can repair damaged or aged parts of the body.

This therapy is part of a fast-growing field known as "regenerative medicine."

Mr. Cox's article details how this works. He has actually had his heart muscle cells rejuvenated.

I'll try to simplify how this works. Medical researchers use a person's skin cells and reproduce them over and over. Then these cells are turned into pluripotent stem cells (induced pluripotent stem cells, or iPSCs) by genetically modifying them until they exactly mirror the embryonic stem cells life starts from.

These new propagated cells are called "immortal" because they don't age. Without getting too technical, the cells don't age because the researchers can stop the loss of telomerase genes by keeping them active, which causes them to constantly reset, which stops the aging process. Why this is important is because at birth each of our cells has only 120 telomeres per chromosome. When a cell depletes its supply of telomeres, it can't replicate itself.

Researchers have the ability to program the iPSCs with the genetic code of any cell and create cells that are the same as the cells in any organ or body part. At that point, the cells begin to age normally, but in essence they are biologically young.

Here is where this gets interesting. If those newly formed cells were injected into a person's body, they would theoretically restore the targeted body part in about a year.

Immortality, at least for now, is probably best left for the gods. Someday soon regenerative medicine will bring us one step closer. All this sounds a little like some of the stuff I've seen in science fiction movies. I'm over sixty years old, and I remember when we didn't have a TV or a phone in our house. And now we can run our TVs and houses by using smartphones that just forty years ago were unimaginable.

Think of the possibilities: repair a broken heart, a damaged liver, or a cancer-ridden lung or breast with regenerated new and younger healthy cells.

The stuff of dreams? Maybe.

But one thing that isn't some far-off technology dream, one thing that will extend your life and make you feel younger, one thing that has been scientifically proven to regenerate the cardiovascular system is a plant-based, whole foods diet.

Look, I am not trying to sound like a "veggie preacher," but I know how much money we as a society spend on chasing the fountain of youth. Humankind has always dreamt of immortality.

Eating right won't make it happen, but if you want to live a longer, healthier life, there is a cheap and easy way to do it.

As far as Susan and I are concerned, we have nothing to lose. Susan was given a death sentence. If eating a different way will extend her time by a day or a week or ten years, then I'm in because keeping her around longer is what I dream of at night when I stare up at the stars. Because . . .

Without Susan, I'm not interested in immortality.

Dealing with Mortality
By Jeff Weaver — Feb 11, 2013, 3:36 p.m.

Do you remember when you were eighteen? I do, and I thought I was indestructible, that nothing could harm me. I don't know whether I thought I was going to live forever, but I didn't think I was going to die either. I didn't even consider dying when I enlisted in the Army in 1967, at the height of the Vietnam War. But as we go about living, we learn about death.

Last time, I wrote about immortality; today, I want to speak to our mortality.

I got a text from my sister Jennifer last Monday. She said, "Mom's bedridden now, calling hospice. . . . She isn't going to get any better. She's too weak to get up and down."

My mom has been going downhill for some time. She has advanced Alzheimer's, and recently she had blood clots in her leg that required hospitalization. At her age, eighty-three, it is just too much for her to endure.

I called my dad, but he was too distressed to speak, so I talked to Jennifer and my niece Kelley. I told them I was coming up, but they told me I didn't have to because I had my own worries down here with Susan. That was a truly gracious thought on their part, but I don't think I would have been able to look in the mirror had I stayed home and not spent time with Mom in her last days.

So, I threw some things in a bag and headed up to Myrtle Creek, to the place I still call home. It's a long, fourteen-hour drive, and I had lots of time to think about my mom's life, my life, and of course Susan's life. I thought a lot about my dad and what he must be going through. He and Mom just had their sixty-sixth anniversary. That's a long time to spend with one person.

But time moves ever forward, and it seems like, as I age, time really does fly by. As I drove, I wondered where all of it had gone. I thought about what I wanted to do with my remaining time and all the things I wanted to do with and for Susan.

As I drove, I remembered years ago listening to my dad talk about buying a sailboat and sailing to far-off places, to places in the South Pacific he saw during World War II. Only this time it would be him and Mom taking their sweet time. I remembered Mom talking about going to Europe and visiting Rome and Paris and Athens. My mom was a big dreamer, and she wanted much out of life.

But I think it is the same with most of us: some of our dreams are just dreams. I mean, don't we all dream of things that will never be? That's not such a bad thing though.

As I drove, I thought about what my mom did in her life and the people she touched. I know Mom has had a big impact on a lot of people, many of them the kids who grew up in Myrtle Creek. She managed and taught swimming lessons at the Myrtle Creek swimming pool for many years. She became a member of the Nazarene Church and was very active in church functions. Mom is a breast cancer survivor, and after she fought and won that battle, she became a hospice volunteer and visited hundreds of others as they went through their final days. My mom is a doer.

When I got to Myrtle Creek Tuesday afternoon, she was worse than I thought or maybe worse than I hoped she would be. I was surprised by how many of her grandchildren, great-grandchildren, and great-great-grandchildren were there. Her room was packed with them, and some had traveled thousands of miles just to spend a few more days at her side. It was a tribute to her, and their presence showed how revered Mom was. I was very moved, thrilled, and extremely saddened.

But all that didn't get to me as much as watching my dad did. This was a lot harder on him than I imagined because my dad is such a tough man. I've only once seen him get really emotional—the day his dad died.

I want to stray a little here because I was with my grandfather when he passed, and I will never forget something Grandma said to me while we were waiting for my dad to show up. She said, "For the past several months all your grandfather wanted to do was hold my hand. If I would have known he wanted that, I would have done it a long time ago." Simple regrets; I suspect we all will have them. I'm sure Dad has his.

Now he wants to do things for Mom that he can't. He wants her to eat and drink, but she won't. He wants to make her feel comfortable every minute of the day, but he can't. But that doesn't stop him from trying and fussing over her constantly; he even sleeps on the couch next to her bed so he can be there if she needs anything. Dad is still fighting, and maybe he is still secretly hoping she'll turn the corner and get better . . . but all that fight and hope won't bring her back to what she was even two months ago.

It was hard watching him beat himself up for not doing more for her or for changing her bandages and hurting her when he tries to get her out of bed. I knew how much pain he was in. However, I also saw how much he cares for her. I saw more affection from him for Mom than I ever have. She still has her lucid moments, and she always knows who Dad is. Even though she is at the end of her road and nearing death, I saw them tease each other and even have a few laughs together. I saw a lot of love in that house.

I didn't talk to him about what he's going through other than to let him know everyone was there for him as much as they were for Mom. He is really lucky to have my niece Kelley, who works in the medical field, and my sister-in-law Loretta, whose job is caring for the elderly, around. One thing he won't have to worry about is going through this alone. Our family is big and everyone cares deeply for my folks.

But when it comes to getting through things like this mentally and having to deal with the mortality of the ones you care the most about . . . well, that's a road each of us must travel alone. My dad is finding his way down this road now.

I left Friday, around noon. I felt torn; I wanted to get home to Susan, but I didn't want to leave my home in Oregon and my folks. I went up there because I thought they might need me for something. But really it was me that needed something. I know Mom doesn't recognize me most of the time, but I was hoping she would so I could say goodbye.

When I left no one was there but Mom and Dad and me. I walked over to her bed and said, "Mom, I'm going home."

She reached up and took my hand and smiled at me. "Me too," she said.

I believe at that moment she knew who I was and she knew exactly what she was saying.

As I drove, I knew I would never again hear Mom's soft, comforting voice telling me I would be okay when I was sick or feel the warmth of her shoulder that I had cried on so many times or see the soft, warm glow in her face when she ran her hand through my hair and told me, "Here, let me fix you up," before we walked into church every Sunday. I had to pull off to the side of the road because I started crying so much I couldn't see the lanes.

But later, as I drove, I laughed a little, too. I remembered the time Dad tried to teach her to ride the new BSA motorcycle he had bought her and how she had raced at breakneck speed across the field of barley, escaping the lesson in one piece. And when she crashed his new trail bike into a stone wall—she was okay, but the bike, not so much. The thing I will always remember, and it never fails to bring on a smile, is the smell of smoke and burnt food emanating from the kitchen and Mom telling us, "If it's brown, it's cooking. If it's black, it's done." Boy, we had a lot of "done" food when we were growing up!

I have my regrets that I didn't get to do more for her than I have. And, like they always do, my thoughts then turned back to Susan.

For almost one year now, I've been forced to deal with Susan's mortality. Even though things are looking up for her, there are no guarantees with stage 4 cancer.

I can't guarantee that we'll be able to do all the things Susan and I have dreamed of or put money worries behind us. I know we both will have our regrets at the end. Who doesn't?

Like all mortals, our time here on Earth is limited, and Mom's time is up. She is fortunate to have so many of her loved ones by her side. And I think it's safe to say Susan will never have to worry about being alone when her time is up. Like my mom, Susan has touched many others throughout her life, and she is now teaching us how to fight for every minute of it.

And that may be the best gift Susan will ever give us.

A Sad Day
By Jeff Weaver — Feb 13, 2013, 5:16 p.m.

Yesterday morning my mom, Sandra, passed. She was born in Binghamton, New York, on August 23, 1930. In the last days of her life, she was surrounded by her family, who cared for her right up until the end, just like she cared for us all her adult life . . . with love and compassion.

Susan, Josh, Nicole, and I will leave Friday to attend her service on Saturday. This will be the last journal entry until after February 22, which is the date of Susan's next visit to her oncologist. Both Susan and I are getting more nervous about each new visit. We pray that she is continuing her improvement.

And one more thing: Mom, Godspeed, and you have a safe trip as well. I love you, and all of us here will miss you.

Old Friends, Saying Goodbye, and Surprises
By Jeff Weaver — Feb 18, 2013, 11:16 p.m.

The pastor stood at the pulpit and looked out over the crowd gathered in the Nazarene Church. His eyes moved from one side to the other and from the first row to the back row. Men, women, children, all sat waiting for him to speak.

"We are here to celebrate the life of Sandra Weaver."

And that we did.

Susan, Josh, Nicole, and I made the trip to pay our respects to Mom on Saturday. The church was packed. Many of the people Mom had touched during her life came to say their goodbyes.

Many of my oldest friends were there, and some I hadn't seen in years. They may have been my friends, but they were also my mom's friends. Like all small towns, you end up a part of several families. Everyone pitched in and helped raise each other's kids.

After the service we all gathered to eat and talk and remember.

I spoke to as many as I could. I wanted to thank them for being my mom's friend and for coming to celebrate her life. I learned a few things about Mom that I didn't know. Like how she would go pick up members of the church who needed rides to church services or functions. And how much time she spent with people who needed a helping hand with household chores or shopping . . . anything they needed, Mom was there for them. I guess I shouldn't have been so surprised because as I said before, Mom was a doer.

My mom was really close with her older sister, Billy, and her niece and nephew, Linda and Jimmy. I know how much Mom looked up to Billy and how much she admired Linda and Jimmy because both were very accomplished and talented kids who grew up to be accomplished people. In fact, my sister Jennifer and I were in a sort of competition with them all our lives. As a result, I have always followed their lives and even envied them. I have, in many ways, lived in their rather large shadows because I know how much Mom thought of them.

When I had a chance to talk to Jimmy, I told him about how many times Mom would tell me about all his athletic feats, his musical prowess, and his business successes and how she compared me to him all my life. We both had a good chuckle over that. I also told him I never minded it either. I know Jimmy loved my mom.

Then I had a conversation with Linda. She was one of Mom's favorite people. Linda is very smart and beautiful; in fact, she was a professional model for many years. Linda is one of the nicest people I have ever met. She has a graciousness that you don't often encounter. Anyway, I told Linda how much Mom cared for her and how Jennifer and I sometimes felt that we lived in her and Jimmy's shadows. I told her that I sometimes was a little jealous of them because of the praise Mom heaped on them. And I confessed that praise wasn't something we heard much of growing up, and I don't ever remember either of us being told we had done well.

Then, Linda told me something that really surprised me. She said her mom was very hard on her and never complimented her either. And that her relationship with her mom was strained and difficult at times.

I guess because we were in a church it was okay to be confessional. Linda and I talked a lot about my relationship with my dad and how I have lived my whole life trying to please him and how I have been a disappointment to him. I don't want to get too much into this, but I will say this is a big deal to me because my dad was my hero when I was growing up and he still is.

As things were winding down and we were saying goodbye to everyone, Linda pulled me aside. We walked over to a quiet corner, and she said, "I talked to your dad a minute ago. He told me how proud he was of you for all you have done for Susan." Then she gave me a hug and said, "I thought you should know this because I know how much it means to you."

Like I said, we came to say goodbye to Mom and to celebrate her life. And in doing so I learned how much my mom had done for others and, to my surprise, I learned that I had finally done something to make my dad proud of me.

I don't typically do things for a pat on the back, but let me tell you this: getting a pat on the back from your hero does feel pretty damn good, even when it's a secondhand pat.

The $10,000 Bet
By Jeff Weaver — Feb 24, 2013, 2:24 p.m.
Dr. Kashani said, "I'll bet you $10,000. . . ."

That statement was worth every cent of the bet, and if I had the money, I'd match it. So, what am I talking about anyway?

What a difference one year makes.

One year ago our lives were altered forever when we found out Susan had cancer. We heard her doctor say there was no cure and no hope of her living a long, peaceful life. We heard she was terminal, and the hope was that her team of doctors would be able to extend her life for a few more years. Imagine being forty-eight years old and in the prime of your life, and then you hear that you are going to die.

One year ago no bets were made that day, no promises, no guarantees, and, to tell the truth, no words of real hope. The only positive thing we heard was that her doctors would do everything they could to make sure Susan would be as comfortable as they could make her for as long as they could. Even those kind words were sobering.

Friday, Susan and I met with her oncologist to review the last three months and to get an update on her lab work. As I've said before, Dr. Kashani is a really nice man and he can't hide his emotions—and that's putting it mildly!

After he examined Susan, he said, "I want to show you something." As he pulled up her charts, he told her how proud he was of her. Then he said, "Look at this, 44.2."

Susan seemed kind of disappointed and told him she was hoping to see 39 because she wants to be normal again. He told her that if she is within 5 percentage points on either side of 39, that is considered to be normal. He even drew a bell curve on the whiteboard to illustrate what he meant. He said she is so close now: 5 percent is 2 points, so if her numbers go down just 3 more points, she will be within the margin.

So, let's get back to the bet. Dr. Kashani is elated with how Susan is responding and how great she looks. He said, "I would be willing to bet $10,000 that no one would know you're a cancer patient." He also said she was more likely to outlive him because of some health issues he has. Without hesitation, Susan told him he should look into making a few changes in his diet and offered to buy him the *Forks Over Knives* book and video.

I, too, love how Susan looks, and I especially love her hair. But there is something else that makes her beauty shine through. And that is her newfound inner strength. I see it in her eyes. She has a kind of glow about her now that's hard to describe but easy to see. I see how hard she fights every single day, and I know that in and of itself sets her apart.

Susan is not out of the woods yet, and we know cancer is a fierce adversary. Look, the odds of cancer patients who are at stage 4 surviving are around 10 percent. That's not a very good bet.

Susan *is* an amazing woman and a fierce warrior as well, and I'm here to tell you . . .

Don't bet against her!

Great News: Markers Down Again
By Jeff Weaver — Mar 5, 2013, 12:51 p.m.
I wanted to share the news Susan got last night. In an email from her oncologist, he wanted to tell her that her markers as of February 28 were . . . DRUM ROLL, PLEASE:

37

That means from January 3, when they were 44.2, they have gone down enough to put her in the normal range. Needless to say, Susan was very excited. But her test also revealed something I am worried about.

Her estrogen levels have more than doubled since December. Her doctor told her not to fret over that. RIGHT! One thing that cancer gives you is a healthy dose of anxiety. It's the gift that, unfortunately, keeps on giving.

Because Susan's cancers (remember, she has two separate types) are estrogen based and she is on an anti-estrogen therapy regimen, something is causing the rapid rise in those numbers. So, I have to think diet must be playing a part in this. From everything I've read, some foods replicate estrogen when consumed and some foods help the body produce more of the hormone. I thought I was doing everything to make sure Susan wasn't eating anything that would do this.

For the next few days, I will be going over everything she has eaten in the past couple months to see if there is anything I have missed. Because she has been doing so well, I've tried to expand her diet a little by adding a few more foods. But I think until I figure this out we will go back to the basics. Well, basics for us: plenty of leafy greens, brightly colored veggies, fresh fruits and berries, nuts, and legumes. Thankfully, we have a great certified organic farmers market just a couple miles from here that has nearly everything we need.

For now, we will celebrate the latest good news and I will make sure we thank Susan's medical team and God for helping us get to this point.

New Studies and Lifestyle Changes
By Jeff Weaver — Mar 29, 2013, 12:32 p.m.
It's been a hectic and busy couple weeks. We have been doing a lot of moving. Three weeks ago I started moving into a new office in downtown LA. It is located right smack in the middle of Korea Town. I have no clue as to what other kinds of businesses are around us because most of the signage is in Korean. Anyway, all of our stuff for the office was in storage in San Dimas, and sure enough the things we needed were in the back of the units. But that was a piece of cake compared to moving all the heavy furniture and equipment into the office, which is on the sixth floor.

Then, the day after moving the office, Susan and I helped Nicole move to her new digs in Huntington Beach. Sadly, she is moving because she and Kevin have decided it was in their best interest to part ways. This is hard on everyone, including Susan, because we really like Kevin. But Susan is doing her best to support Nicki any way she can. I have to say, Susan is a great mother and seems to know just the right words and when to say them.

But the biggest thing for us is that my commute can be nearly two hours each way to LA (love the traffic down there—not!), and I'm in the office ten to twelve hours a day. That means Susan has to do all the cooking now. I am superstressed that she isn't getting enough rest because cooking like we do takes time. And I hardly get to see her because by the time I get home all I do is eat and then it's bedtime.

On Wednesday I finally had a moment to do a little reading and caught up on a few new studies.

Here are the highlights.

An article on the Oncology Practice website dealt with the side effects of radiation therapy on breast cancer patients (March 20, 2013). The study's researchers tracked women over a span of forty-three years and found that the women were more likely to suffer a major ischemic stroke, the most common type of stroke, because of the frequency and dosage of their traditional radiation treatments.

They found the risk began to increase within the first five years of treatment and continued to increase for at least twenty years.

Forty-four percent of breast cancer patients suffered "major coronary events" in the first 10 years after their diagnosis; 33 percent of events occurred 10 to 19 years after diagnosis, and 23 percent occurred 20 or more years later. Fifty-four percent of all the patients who had had a "major coronary event" died of ischemic heart disease.

Fifty-four percent. That's a pretty big deal. Now I'm glad that Susan didn't have radiation therapy treatments.

Another study I read discussed women who have mastectomies. In many cases women choose to have a double mastectomy, hoping to eliminate the risk of cancer in a healthy breast even when their cancer is confined to one breast. The rate of contralateral prophylactic mastectomies (CPMs) is rising. CPM just means having both breasts removed.

In an analysis of overall survival of patients with stages 1 to 3 of invasive breast cancer, there was no significant difference in survival rates of patients who underwent a CPM compared with those who had only one breast removed regardless of whether they had received neoadjuvant chemotherapy.

And this, as reported on the Fox News website in the Health section: new research has found more than twice the number of genetic variations associated with breast, prostate, and ovarian cancer (March 27, 2013). This is important because healthcare practitioners now will have more ways to screen at-risk patients, which will lead to better drugs and treatment methods.

The study involved two hundred thousand people. Researchers identified seventy-four gene changes for the three hormone-related cancers.

These new findings will make it possible for drug companies to create compounds that work more effectively. The article stated that "scientists stressed that genes were just one side of a complex mix of factors leading to cancer" and "that lifestyle and environmental risks act in concert with the genetics. It is not one or the other—it is always both together."

I saw another article on the Fox News website in the Health section about how lifestyle and attitude play a big role in the recovery process of cancer patients and anyone with a major illness (Fox News, March 26, 2013).

In 2009, a forty-year-old woman, Ms. Russo, was diagnosed with stage 3 colorectal cancer. By following the practices of health and wellness expert Deepak Chopra, she changed her attitude and her diet to a healthier one, and beat her cancer.

Here are Chopra's six tips to maintaining wellness (I think this is good for us all, sick or not):

Set goals and priorities. "[E]stablish a baseline health status and decide where you want to be, and what it's going to take in terms of lifestyle, also in terms of standard treatment."

Get rid of processed foods. Basically, this means throwing out food that is "processed, refined, or manufactured . . . anything that comes in a can or label." If you do buy canned or packaged products, learn to read labels so you can eliminate foods with harmful ingredients.

Practice meditation and visualization. "Russo said when she got sick, she would sit outside and visualize the sun, with all her kids home and a big swimming pool—and this is what they would do when she was healthy."

"Visualization actually changes your behavior. . . . If you visualize a healthy, energetic, joyful body, and a quiet, restful mind, then that in itself will influence how you do other things."

Express your emotions. "It's not that you have to think positively all the time," Chopra said. "You have to get in touch with your emotions. You have to share them with somebody that you love. . . . You have to express them, because if you repress emotions, that creates its own biology, too." He added, "You have to talk about your problems—tell people if you are happy, scared, sad or angry."

Resist alienating yourself. "You need to connect with peace, harmony, laughter, and love—it's as simple as that."

Learn the science of self-repair. "Russo said she is a different person now—she's more tolerant—and she does not believe her cancer will ever come back."

Four years later, Ms. Russo is cancer free.

I know this sort of thing works. When I was diagnosed, I stayed positive, made changes in my life, and refused to give in to cancer. I didn't talk about it with others very much, and if I did, I made light of my condition. As for Susan, you all know what we have done and you have read about her miraculous recovery . . . so far, anyway. (We also believe in not being too cocky or patting ourselves on the back too soon.)

All those steps help. After reading them, I think Susan and I need to periodically do an assessment to make sure we have priorities in order. One thing I have to do fast is adjust to my new schedule. I told her yesterday that I felt really guilty because I couldn't take care of her like I have been.

I feel strongly that rest is a big deal for her, and I hate not seeing her more. (Thank God for text messaging. I think it is the best thing they have invented since . . . well, sliced bread.) When I was home more, I watched her like a hawk, always checking on how tired she was and making sure she ate all the right things, and I tried to make sure her mind was in the right place. Of course, a big reason why I hate not being home more is because Susan is my favorite person and I can't think of a single person on this earth I would rather spend my time with.

Finally, this Sunday is Easter, and I'll be in church. Because of the scare we've had with Susan and my mother's passing, celebrating the resurrection means more to me now.

Learning to Live with Cancer: Fighting Fatigue
By Jeff Weaver — Apr 13, 2013, 5:53 p.m.

It's a scary deal when you face an advanced disease with little hope of surviving it. You don't know what to expect or how to deal with the wide range of problems, from financial issues to the physical demands and, maybe scariest of all, the emotional stress that you face. The unknowns wear you down.

It takes strength to fight cancer. It takes dedication, a plan of attack both medically and mentally, as well as lifestyle choices. And it takes support from everyone you know.

One of the hardest things to overcome for anyone is how to handle fatigue and how to push through those times when it starts to get the best of you.

This week has been a rough week for Susan. Two weeks ago she had all three of her treatments on the same day, and the side effects this time are bad. One night last weekend when we went to bed, she was in a lot of pain. Her bones ached and her joints hurt so bad she had to take prescription pain medication (for her, that's bad!). She couldn't sleep because of severe hot flashes. I reached over and put my hand on her side to comfort her, and she was soaking wet from sweating.

Then she said something that worried me. "I don't want to do this anymore. It's not worth this. I want to stop taking the treatments. What's the use if I'm going to feel like this the rest of my life? Besides, how long do I have because everything says the treatments are going to kill me anyway? I just want my old life back."

Now sometimes I hear similar questions from her, and I know they are rhetorical, not literal. But this time was different. And you know what? These are fair questions to ask.

Cancer is wearing her out. The treatments and the constant need to fight are grinding away at her willpower every day. Now, I know what you're thinking: she's getting better, her numbers are way down, her doctors are amazed at her progress. All true, but here's the deal. She knows the reason why her doctors told her she will never be "cured" is because they can't guarantee that, and she knows that only 10 percent of people who are stage 4 cancer survive longer than five years.

Susan has been getting more pessimistic, partly because she has never had to deal with a long-term medical issue. This kind of mental fatigue can be as deadly as the disease.

I have done my best to reassure her that she will win this battle. But then we have a week like this one, and even my optimism takes a dip.

Why is it that when some well-known person dies, it can really get to us? This week Roger Ebert lost his long battle with cancer. Both Susan and I were saddened and a little shaken because we have been following his progress and because, like Susan, he too was on a plant-based diet. Just two days before his death he announced plans for what he would do going forward. Consequently, I had to reassure Susan that his situation was very different from hers.

Then, on Wednesday our landlord sent me a text saying she needed to talk to us. She came over to inform us that we had to move. Her sister lost her house and needs a place to live. I understand the landlord is looking out for her sister, but it still sucks and adds a lot of additional stress we don't need right now because we don't have any place to go or the extra money it takes to move. While she was giving us our notice, she told us her other sister, who has been fighting stage 3 cancer, found out last week that her cancer is back and it looks pretty bad for her. We don't know her sister, and we feel for her, but the news of her recurrence was one more reminder of how cancer works.

And to top off an otherwise crappy week, I read an update for Drew Hilliard, the young Navy lieutenant. A month or so ago his doctors found a suspicious spot on a scan, so he had a follow-up scan done last week. The news was not good. The spots have grown in size, so now he has to have surgery and maybe chemo. Drew is young and has a healthy lifestyle. We have been following his progress, and this news hit both of us hard because we feel a special connection to Drew. So, now Susan has more questions and more doubt and less hope.

I can feel the hope she has built up lately draining from her every time she hears about someone who has a recurrence. And there is something else that worries me. Since I'm back to work and because I don't get home until late, Susan never gets to rest. She comes home and has to do the cooking. She is on her feet at four forty-five in the morning and goes until eight o'clock at night. Physical fatigue is a big deal when you're fighting cancer because it weakens the immune system and can increase inflammation in the cells, but maybe worse, it breaks down your resolve and weakens you mentally.

It's this mental fatigue I'm starting to get most concerned about. Many studies have shown that people who have a positive outlook have better outcomes in almost every aspect of life, while other studies show that people with negative attitudes have more medical, financial, and emotional trouble. Plus, I know from personal experience when you become negative you start looking for and expecting bad things to happen. It becomes like a self-fulfilling prophecy, and it's a vicious circle that's hard to break out of.

With everything I have personally been through lately, mental fatigue has become a problem for me, too. I find I have less drive, less motivation to write and exercise, less will to be patient with people—and that includes my family, and that's not fair or right. I "snap" far too easily; my language gets rough at times. I have to fight feeling bitter about our situation.

Just this week I struggled to keep my emotions in check. Twice I couldn't hold back the tears when I thought of how bad Susan hurts and what life would be like if she wasn't here. Yes, I know, suck it up. And I do, but I'm telling you it's getting harder to stay positive. Mostly, all this is the result of outside events and not Susan's cancer. But her cancer is the elephant that is always in the room.

One thing we have talked about is how important it is to stay focused on our personal plan to fight her cancer. She wants to make sure she gets enough raw whole foods so she can take advantage of all the cancer-fighting compounds in the foods she eats. And she wants to make sure she is not eating anything that will fuel her cancer.

I have to try to stay as positive as I can. That has always been my job: be Mr. Positive even when things go haywire. I have always been Susan's biggest cheerleader when it comes to career and her art, but now I have to channel some of that toward her mental fight.

And I see a sort of mental fatigue in her friends as well. Everyone has their own daily struggles and only so much energy to spread around.

Make no mistake, Susan is one tough lady. I am amazed and inspired by her daily. But even the toughest can be beaten or worn down by the kind of fight she is engaged in.

Life is a series of good and bad things, and when the bad comes it takes strength to get through to a better place.

And it takes willpower . . . but that's a topic for another day.

The New Normal
By Jeff Weaver — May 18, 2013, 6:27 p.m.

Cancer changes everything. It changes how body cells grow—it causes them to grow bigger and faster than normal cells. Then, like an alien mutant army, the cancerous cells divide rapidly, creating more diseased cells that continue to grow and divide at an ever-increasing rate. As this mutant army of cancer cells takes over the body, it, like all armies, must be fed. The cancer cells consume more and more of the nutrients in the blood stream, and the normal cells actually starve, until the host eventually dies. Cancer changes how you go about your everyday tasks, how you eat, how you sleep, how you think . . . in essence, how you live. And it also changes everything for the ones who stand by the patient's side in the fight.

Susan keeps saying she just wants to go back to being a normal person.

Normal. Sounds like a simple enough desire.

But cancer also changes what normal is. What's normal for Susan is not normal for me or Josh or Nicole. However, we all must adapt to her new normal. And we must accept that none of us is ever going back to what was normal before Susan was told she had maybe five years to live. Or, put another way, before her death sentence—strong words, huh? Yes, but true words, and that is why cancer changes everything.

Normal for Susan these days is the constant fear that every new pain or ache is a sign *it* is back.

Remember, when we last saw her doctor, her CA 27-29 cancer markers were 37. Normal. Well, we saw her oncologist, Dr. Kashani, this Wednesday. We were anxious to find out what the numbers were this time.

Dr. Kashani was late, but when he finally came into the exam room, he nearly blurted out, "Have you seen your markers?" We knew from his reaction and the huge smile on his face the news was good. "Here, let me show you," as he pulled up her chart. "Look at this, 36.7. That's fantastic, that's a 1200 percent improvement," he said, pointing to the beginning of the graph.

He told us how proud he is of her; he called her his "miracle girl." I watched Susan's face closely as Dr. Kashani showed her the graph and told her how well she was doing. When she heard 36.7 her face lit up. She asked, "Does this mean I can stop my treatments now?" He looked at me and then at her and said, "No, you have to have them for the rest of your life."

Her smile disappeared and a look of real disappointment replaced it. That look caused a hurt to rush from my head to my toes. It struck me that she just got great news, yet she wasn't jumping up and down with joy. She really hurts. And she knows that the pain is now from her treatments, and so long as she has to have them, she will continue to hurt every single minute of every day . . . for the rest of her life.

We talked about her treatments, and she nearly begged him to take her off of them. One thing about Dr. Kashani is that he is such a nice man, and he wants Susan to be comfortable, so he actually considered granting her wish. They discussed the pros and cons.

He was dancing around the words, so I felt compelled to frame the discussion. I looked into her eyes and said, "Look, here's the deal. You can go off the treatments, but most likely your cancer will come back and kill you, or you can deal with the pain from the treatments and live. Personally, I want you to stick around, but this is your call."

Now, I am not overdoing this. This was a serious conversation held in earnest. We decided that Susan would visit a specialist to see what can be done about her wrists, and Dr. Kashani gave her a prescription to try to control the hot flashes. And he allowed more time between treatments to see if that would help.

I told Dr. Kashani I knew how hard this kind of conversation had to be for him. He stopped talking for a minute, and then told us about a young thirty-year-old mother of three who was also his patient. He said a few months ago he told her she was stage 4 and she had only a short time to live. On her next visit she brought in a picture of her three kids, showed it to him, and asked him how she was to tell them she wouldn't live to see them grow up. He told her he didn't know the answer to that, but not to give up because miracles happen. Then he told this young mom about Susan and how she had gotten the same news. He told her that Susan never gave up and made a lot of lifestyle changes and is now his "miracle girl." He really *is* proud of her!

Dr. Kashani paused, and then said something that really touched me. "I hate telling people they're going to die. It's the worst thing I have to do, and I never get used to it. If I could go to God and ask one question, it would be, Why do I have to tell people this . . . why?"

Pretty powerful stuff. Before he left the room he shook our hands and thanked us several times, as if we were the ones curing Susan. We know we are doing our part, but what we do is only a piece of the puzzle of which he is a vital part, and we told him so. When he was gone Susan and I stood and held each other for a time and she said, "I just wish I could be normal again."

All I could say is, "Baby, you are normal, the numbers say so."

This, I'm afraid, is the new normal for us. This is one way cancer has changed us.

Choices and Moving
By Jeff Weaver — Jun 1, 2013, 10:36 a.m.

Yesterday Susan saw the specialist about her wrists and neck. And my suspicions were correct. The severe pain in her wrists is a tendon issue. Apparently, this type of injury is common, and the only remedy is not to use her hands to lift things, and even then that may not help. This type of injury is a crapshoot because they don't know much about it or how to alleviate the pain or the problem. The doctor gave her cortisone shots in both wrists to see if that would help. He also told her she should refrain from lifting. But that is a problem.

Susan's job as a merchandiser requires lots of lifting; in fact, she can't do her job without it. This puts her in a sort of a catch-22. I am afraid of having her take even more time off because Macy's has been eliminating full-time positions. Susan is a great employee and does a fantastic job for Macy's, but if she's not there, well, she has no value to them, and consequently she runs the risk of losing her full-time status, or worse.

She needs her job because of the insurance. Without that, we would be in a world of hurt financially because we can't afford to pay the premiums for private insurance. Plus, we have to make sure she builds up enough goodwill with the company in case she has a recurrence, which would most certainly require additional time off.

You see where I'm going with this, right? Susan is in a difficult situation. It boils down to this: work and suffer the pain, or take time off and risk losing her job. Some choice, huh?

One thing Susan and I talk about is managing the side effects of the drugs she's on. They have a cumulative effect, so this is just the start of these types of problems. We can only hope these problems are minimal and that she can make it through her treatments long enough to hear the magic words, "We have a new drug that will cure you."

Oh, on the moving thing. We found a place in Brea, up Carbon Canyon Road. Our place is right on the edge of the Chino Hills State Park. The view from the backyard is rolling hills and deep canyons and a few rattlesnakes, but not many houses or people.

This will be our sixth move in twelve years! And it will, hopefully, be the last one for a long time.

One thing Susan told me a while back was that she wanted her own home again. Well, her prayers have been answered and again we are indebted to the kindness of others.

The next couple weeks will be hectic. I'm working three different jobs now and put in over twelve hours every day and drive three hours to and from work, so my time is limited. Susan will take some vacation time to finish packing, and I'll take a couple days off to do the move.

Last weekend we went through some of our "treasures" and of course we found lots of old photos and old cards and things the kids made in school. That is always an emotional thing. First, it's "oh, honey, look at this," and then it's do we keep it or part with it?

But we will manage this like we always do. One thing I can tell you is that we are getting pretty damn good at "surviving" life.

Cancer has had such a negative impact on our life, first with me when it stopped me in my tracks and ruined my career and forced me in other directions. Now Susan's cancer is forcing new and equally tough choices and challenges on us.

But in a couple weeks . . . Susan can finally hang her pictures on her own walls.

Learning to Live with Cancer: Shoes and Elephants
By Jeff Weaver — Jul 9, 2013, 11:56 a.m.

We all have heard the clichés "waiting for the other shoe to drop" and "the elephant in the room." But I wonder whether their meanings have been diluted because of overuse or misuse.

What I mean is we hear these sayings so often we tend not to grasp their true meanings. I'm as guilty of using these clichés as anyone. We kind of get what the speaker is trying to convey, but the impact or importance is lost.

Susan is in a constant state of worry, waiting for the other shoe to drop, and it's my guess it goes far beyond worry. Even though she hides it most of the time, I know it's there, like the elephant in the room. And I know how terrified she is.

Susan said something to me a couple nights ago that really worries me. I have learned not to take her premonitions lightly. I did that in the months before she was diagnosed, and I won't make that mistake again.

We were in the kitchen putting together our lunches for the next day, and she said, "Jeffery, we need to talk."

The hair on the back of my neck stands up when I hear "Jeffery." It usually means I'm in big trouble or there is big trouble. So, I waited for the shoe.

"I think you better prepare yourself for bad news."

I asked her why.

She told me she has had a pain deep in her thigh, right below her pelvic bone, where they originally found her cancer. It was one of the biggest worries her team of doctors had. I have tried to reassure her it's just some sort of muscle pain, maybe an injury from work or another side effect from the drugs. But the elephant, in our case, cancer, is never far away. With elephants, it's never wise to ignore them because with one step they can . . . well, I don't need to finish that sentence.

I reminded her how well she is doing, how excited her doctor is with her progress, and how her markers are now normal. But I didn't or couldn't take away the fear she felt or quiet that voice in her that's telling her something is wrong.

She emailed her doctor, and he has scheduled her for a series of X-rays. I think she will have them done this week.

I have mentioned this before, but it bears repeating. Susan is losing her confidence about her long-term prognosis. She sees the test results and is grateful and happy. She knows she has the best medical care and a highly skilled and caring physician in Dr. Kashani. But the fact is, the odds of surviving long term because she is at stage 4 are not very good, and that is the elephant that follows her everywhere and is always in the room with her. It takes up a lot of space.

I know Susan feels snakebit (yes, I used another cliché), but I also know she is a fighter. I marvel at her determination and strength.

I think this pain is nothing to worry about. But I am sure she will worry until she has answers.

And I am sure that every new pain will bring new worries. Susan and I have learned a lot, and we don't kid ourselves anymore.

We are learning how to sidestep falling shoes and how to live with elephants.

Quick Update
By Jeff Weaver — Jul 11, 2013, 3:30 p.m.
Susan has gotten a very fast response from Dr. Kashani on the X-rays she had done. He said there was no evidence of fractures. No joint disease and no significant soft tissue abnormality. He didn't say what he thought the pain in her thigh was. It's my guess it is some sort of nerve thing going on. We see him next month, and we should get a better idea then. For now, we can breathe a sigh of relief . . . at least until the next pain or threat comes along.

One more thing I would like to say. I've been watching Susan very closely for some time. I look for signs that things are not normal. I watch to see how she is holding up mentally and physically. I watch to make sure she isn't getting too run down. And I watch how she reacts to everyday life. It's that part I am most fascinated with. I am witnessing a dramatic evolution in her, and it is fascinating and exciting and wondrous all at the same time.

What I am witnessing now is something extraordinary, and I love who she is evolving into.

How Sweet It Is
By Jeff Weaver — Oct 16, 2013, 11:27 a.m.
It's been a few months since I wrote an update. I've been busy working three jobs, from seven in the morning to nine or ten at night seven days a week, plus we started some major remodeling work on the house. Frankly, I'm tired, and so I stopped writing almost entirely and I find myself losing focus. For most of us, it is hard to sort out what's really important in life and get our priorities straight. I was better at this when I was younger . . . oh, to be thirty-two again.

For the past couple months, I've been working more hours for Vinyl Window Broker. We are in the home improvement industry. It's been interesting because I do estimates for folks who want to remodel their homes. I spend two to three hours visiting with them, and the biggest hurdle I face is helping these folks determine what their most important project is.

I have been wearing a pink wristband since Susan was diagnosed, and everyone I meet asks me about it. I tell them about the battle Susan is fighting and how we have made major changes in our lifestyle and especially our diet. They are genuinely moved by her story, and most of them think that diet is a big deal. But in the next breath they say, "I don't think I would have the willpower to do that."

I've learned not to preach at people, but I do let them know how important I think it is to eat better. I tell them for us it boils down to two choices: life or death.

And then I tell them it isn't easy to be as strict as we are, but we are in a different place, and they don't have to be that restrictive. I add that, by making a few changes now, they may never have to go through what Susan is going through.

Every single homeowner I talk to knows how sincere I am about this, and they ask for advice. I am happy to give it. I have discovered I'm good at helping people make choices, whether it is what project to do on their home or how to revamp their diet, by giving them good information. I tell them to focus on the really important things in life because you never know how long you have.

Yesterday I had to turn in a couple contracts to my office in Tustin. I had a little time to kill, and I found myself turning into the parking lot of Irvine Valley College. It's where I resumed my college education after a forty-year "break." I've met some awesome people there and have made some good friends. But, more importantly, I've had professors who have really inspired me and who have pushed me and prodded me. They gave me knowledge that has allowed me to have the confidence to stretch outside my comfort zone.

I went up to the writing lab and saw Julie Evans. Julie is one of the first writing professors I had, and she was tough and totally awesome! We had a good conversation. She asked how Susan was doing and I gave her the latest news. I got a little emotional, and so did Julie. As I struggled to regain my composure, I realized what was really important to me. I felt a new determination to finish school. So, I went over to the counselor's office and set in motion the coursework to pursue a degree in English with an emphasis in writing.

I needed someone to help me prioritize. I needed information from others to be successful. Because life isn't easy and sometimes making the right choice is hard.

From all my years of experience, I know hard work and determination make things happen. It takes focus to succeed. And I know that hard work, determination, and focus can sometimes bring about miracles.

Last night Susan and I took a twenty-minute drive to Ontario to visit her parents, who are down here to pick up a new motorhome. Susan had her treatments just a few hours earlier, so she wasn't feeling very good.

We had dinner with them and of course talked about diet. Ann is all in, but Martin has his doubts. But I know he approves of what Susan is doing. Like I said, we have learned not to preach; instead, we just let people know what we are doing and why.

The drive back home was a little weird. Susan was hurting because of her treatments and she was sad because she knew she wouldn't see her parents again for a long time. But she was at the same time very happy to have had a few hours with them. Living so far from her parents is hard on Susan, and I know it's harder on them because she is all they have now.

Before we went to bed Susan checked her email and there was a message from her oncologist, Dr. Kashani. We knew it was important because he had sent it so late in the evening.

Susan looked at me for what seemed like ten minutes. I tried to read her face and my heart started to race. Then she said . . .

"Thirty-two, my markers are thirty-two." She paused, smiled, and then took a deep breath. "They were 36.7 last time."

Thirty-nine is normal, so this is really great news. We high-fived each other.

Dr. Kashani is right. Susan is a miracle girl. I am so proud of her.

How sweet it is to be thirty-two again.

Learning to Live with Cancer: Being Aware
By Jeff Weaver — Nov 5, 2013, 5:20 p.m.

Breast Cancer Awareness Month just ended. I saw lots of news stories about breast cancer on TV, on my computer, and in the papers. I saw feel-good stories about heroic survivors and heart-wrenching pieces about families whose lives have been turned upside down. There were hundreds of walks and runs and other types of fund-raisers that raised tens of millions of dollars to help finish the fight. Everywhere I turned something was there to bring the fight against breast cancer to the forefront.

But there was something missing in all this. And it's something I think is important: I didn't see a single piece designed to educate people on what they should do or say and what they shouldn't when they are around a cancer patient who is fighting for her life.

How many of you would wave a shot of whiskey under an alcoholic's nose and try to get that person to take a drink? Would you offer a candy bar to a diabetic? Or serve seafood to someone who is allergic to it? Would you take a person dying of cancer to see Margaret Edson's Pulitzer Prize–winning play *Wit*? *Wit* is about a woman dying of cancer, and it is as close to being there as you can get; extraordinarily moving. I highly recommend watching the HBO version. But what if you are doing something similar without knowing it?

I'm pretty tuned in to this sort of thing. One of my new pet peeves is when people try to get Susan to eat foods they know are not on her diet. I don't think they really understand what she is up against, or they don't believe what she is doing will make that big a difference, or they are well meaning and think "just this once won't hurt." Or maybe they see how good she looks and think she is out of danger.

Before I continue, it's important to remember metastatic cancer is incurable. Once cancer moves from the site of origin and attaches to other organs, or spreads throughout the lymph system or into the bones, the chance of survival is less than 10 percent. What doctors do for stage 4 cancer patients is try to extend their lives for a few years.

Okay, back to the point. I see people offer Susan all sort of treats or foods. I hear them tell her it won't hurt her. I even see this in my own house. Our son sometimes teases Susan with a slice of pizza, or ice cream, or some other goodie. Susan and I have dropped a few hints, and he is getting better. Well, there were the chocolate chip cookies he made for himself last week and then left on the counter where Susan could see and smell them. She finally told him to get them out of her sight.

This week I recorded an HBO documentary called *Mondays at Racine*, which is about two women in Racine, New York, who own a hair salon and spa, and one Monday every month cancer patients can go in and get any service free of charge. I thought it would be inspirational. What I didn't do was preview the program. A few nights ago Susan and I watched it. The first thing they showed was a woman who was just starting her fight against breast cancer and who had had two chemo treatments. She was in the shower and her hair was falling out, and then the film showed her in the beauty salon breaking down before she had her hair cut. The next second it showed a woman who has been fighting cancer for ten years— and she looked like it, too—and she and her husband were sitting at a table. He was drinking beer and making hamburgers, and she started talking about the emotional distress she has been through. She said that her doctors were trying to make her as comfortable as possible before cancer took her and that they knew she was in pain, but she felt they didn't see the real picture when she walked out of the hospital and had to suffer through her disease alone at home. Right then, I knew this was a big mistake. Before I could turn off the program, Susan told me to turn it off. I heard a little anger in her tone.

How could I be so damn insensitive? Why didn't I check the content to see whether the program was something Susan would want to see? So, rather than inspire us with something uplifting, I had thrown ice water on our evening. Worse yet, it was another reminder of what she was up against, and that got to her.

Thursday was Halloween, and Susan's coworkers had a potluck.

She took a kale salad. Later that night she told me something that surprised me. She said that when she walked into the room all her friends were gathered around eating goodies, laughing, and having a great time. She said it smelled so good. Then she realized there wasn't anything she could eat and suddenly she felt like an outsider. She had to leave because she was so upset—not at her friends, by the way. She went into a breakroom and sat by herself and cried.

Her coworkers didn't mean to disenfranchise her; they really care for her. But at that moment that's how she felt and was reminded she is not "normal." It was another reminder that her life has been completely altered and she may never be the same again.

Lately, I have had a strong desire to do something that will make a difference in the war on cancer. I read that Drew Hilliard, the young naval officer I've mentioned before, raised over seventeen thousand dollars in a fund-raiser. I read about all the work Noreen Frasier does with her foundation, and this month I saw dozens of stories about young cancer patients raising thousands of dollars.

Because I have had my own long, tough fight with cancer and now watch Susan in her heroic battle, I believe I have a unique perspective on what cancer patients and their families go through. One thing I would like to be able to do is educate folks on some simple but thoughtful things they can do to help a person who is fighting cancer.

If a friend or family member has been diagnosed with cancer, do things with them or for them that you know will cheer them up. Make sure to have a few laughs, too, because laughter is truly medicine and studies have verified it.

One thing that is so important is not to disappear because you are uncomfortable around them or don't know how to talk to them. Just be sensitive about what you say and always stay positive. That is especially true if they have advanced cancer and the prognosis isn't good because people who believe they are dying think much differently about life and death.

If your friend is on a special diet and it seems restrictive or odd to you, it is never okay to tell them "it's okay to cheat just this once" or "don't deprive yourself" of foods they used to eat. Remember, they aren't trying to lose a couple pounds—they are fighting to live. If you want to take them out to dinner, check the menu first to see whether there are healthy dishes that aren't loaded with sugar and salt. That way they will be able to have a good time and you will feel like you are helping them fight cancer.

Please don't offer to buy any alcoholic drinks because that stuff is at the top of the DO NOT HAVE list. Last, I think it is important to give them a big hug now and again. And don't forget to tell them you are praying for them, and then do! Remember they need you more than you know.

In the future around our house: Josh, stop teasing your mom with things you know she can't and won't eat. And as for me, I will be more diligent about my TV viewing. No more war movies or bloody adventure stories and no more stories where the hero or heroine loses the fight against cancer. And I will never again watch my all-time favorite movie, *Sleepless in Seattle*. Even though Susan laughs (and laughter is medicine) at me every time I watch it because I ALWAYS cry at the end. Seriously, what's up with that? I've seen it hundreds of times.

With a little forethought we can all employ a different type of "awareness" in the fight against cancer, and we can do it all year long. By doing these simple things, you will do as much to fight cancer as you would if you had donated money to a charity.

And here is what's in it for you: you will be able to see the payoff in seconds by taking a close look at the face of your friend. You'll see a twinkle in the eyes and a smile, or even tears of joy.

Tis the Season to Give
By Jeff Weaver — Dec 12, 2013, 6:57 p.m.
Here we are in December already, the end of another year. Like most years it's been a mixed bag of good and bad and that always leaves us with as many questions as it does answers. That is especially true in regard to cancer.

I have read several news reports on some very promising new

treatment options and new drug therapies in the pipeline for cancer patients. But I read one disturbing report issued by the World Health Organization's International Agency for Research on Cancer (IARC).

The IARC reported that 14.1 million people were diagnosed with cancer in 2012; that's up from 12.7 million in 2008. And the type of cancer with the largest increase was breast cancer, with 1.7 million new cases just last year and a 20 percent increase since 2008.

These numbers do not reflect cases that are recurrences.

So, what do you think they found to be the cause of such dramatic increases? No surprise here. The report says that the culprit is the adaptation of the Western diet throughout the world.

I am saddened by this news. At this very moment Susan is sitting in a green leather chemo chair getting her two-and-half-hour infusion followed by two other medications; once every three months she has all three treatments on the same day. Sounds like fun, huh? Well, it's not, but there are no alternatives other than to stop her treatments and take her chances.

I'm not sure why, but I'm getting angry. Every week I get two or three calls or emails from people telling me they have a family member or close friend who has been diagnosed with cancer. I feel for all these folks because I know what's in store for them. I hate how cancer can destroy a family emotionally and financially. But again, what can I do? I am not a doctor or a researcher or a good fund-raiser.

I keep wondering if there is something I could do or, even better, something Susan and I could do to help others who hear the awful news, "Sorry, you have cancer."

After all, we certainly have experience in how to fight cancer. We know what to expect and we know the strain it puts on everyone, from patient to family members to friends. We know the pain they will encounter; we know the emotional lows, the fear of the unknown, and all the other things that come with the disease. We know many of the do's and the don'ts when fighting cancer.

One thing that was hard for us both to figure out was all the well-meaning but often conflicting advice we got. Even harder was the lack of accurate information. It's not that that kind of information isn't out there; it's that it's all over the place and it is, many times, sorely outdated or, worse, agenda driven. And that's part of the problem.

Something that is very important to us is information on diet that the medical professionals don't provide. Just this morning Susan saw on TV a piece about a young child who is fighting cancer, and she was sitting in her hospital bed eating pizza. Yikes, can you imagine? If her parents only knew what that pizza is really doing to her.

Last week Susan and I decided to do something about our desire to help others in their fight with cancer. But, even more importantly, we wanted to help so that others never have to go through that fight. Because diet has been such a big part of our focus, it will be a major part of what we do.

We won't try to find a cure for cancer, but by doing something small and vitally important, maybe, just maybe, we can help others fight and hopefully beat cancer.

I have a favor to ask. When you all gather to have that big holiday meal, please say a prayer for those who are fighting cancer and make sure to savor your life and your meal one bite at a time.

Early Christmas Present
By Jeff Weaver — Dec 17, 2013, 3:31 p.m.
Susan and I just finished with her doctor visit. Dr. Kashani was again thrilled with how well she is doing.

He asked Susan if everything is all right, and she told him she is having some issues with lights after dark. To her they are almost neon bright and hurt her eyes. He didn't seem worried and told her he didn't think it was a side effect of her treatments. But he wants her to have a CT scan done of her head, just to be sure nothing is going on. After the holidays she will have one done.

She also told him she can't sleep because of the hot flashes that have been an ongoing problem. Once again she wanted to know if she could stop the Lupron treatments. He said she really shouldn't.

He is going to order a couple tests to see what her estrogen production is like. If he can, he said he might take her off Lupron for a while and see how she responds. I'm on the side of *if it's working stay the course.* But I'm not the one who has to live with the side effects.

Her markers are still at 32. So, everything is going better than we ever would have dreamed.

Susan will stay the course until her next visit in three months. Then Dr. Kashani will see whether he can take her off Lupron. He is so optimistic now, he told us he feels strongly that she is going to beat cancer.

As we left he wished us a Merry Christmas and he hoped we didn't mind because he got in hot water for saying it to a patient who was offended by that. We told him it was fine by us, and with that, Susan hugged him and I shook his hand and we headed home.

And for us, hearing her markers are still 32, well, that was the best holiday greeting ever.

Stressing About Recurrence
By Jeff Weaver — Jan 2, 2014, 10:34am
Ah stress. It goes hand in hand with cancer.

It never really leaves you once you have been diagnosed with advanced cancer. There are a couple reasons: (1) you never want to go through the treatments again because they just aren't fun, and (2) if you have a recurrence, the fight is much tougher the second time around. As I've mentioned before, cancer never really leaves your system, and while it is dormant, it is learning how to fight the body's defense systems and the drugs that were used the first time. And when it learns how to fight back, it does so with a vengeance.

Susan has been having vision problems, so Dr. Kashani ordered a CT scan of her head. He wants to make sure everything is okay.

She is having the scan done today, and we hope to know something in a few days. Her stress level will go up until she finds out what if anything is going on.

As I've mentioned before, it has been proven that a positive attitude and willpower are huge when one is trying to beat cancer. And stress is one of the things a cancer patient needs to try to eliminate because it breaks down the body's ability to defend itself.

I haven't written about this, but I think it's time to address it here. Susan gets irritated with me because she feels like I divulge too much information sometimes. She told me the other day that she feels like I try to make her into a poster child for the fight against cancer.

Truth be told, I do. But here is the deal: I believe that if telling her story helps just one person beat cancer or helps others from ever getting cancer, it is worth sharing her story, warts and all.

And while I'm at it, there is something else on my mind and it has to do with recurrence and the stress of worrying about it, especially if the cancer moves to the brain. Once it goes there the fight is exponentially harder.

I'm not talking about Susan now. About four months ago, I started to feel a pain in my neck. I didn't worry about it at the time. I have pain all over these days, so this was just another one. But it persisted and one day it got really bad. It was bad enough that I was a little scared, so I went to the hospital.

A wonderful doctor, Wendy Coling, examined me. She felt a lump where the lymph nodes are located in my neck. She ordered an ultrasound. It showed that the nodes were enlarged.

She put me on antibiotics because infections are the leading cause of swollen lymph nodes. After I finished the round of antibiotics, the pain hadn't gone away, so she had me do another ultrasound.

This one showed that the nodes had doubled in size. She referred me to a head and neck surgeon. He examined me and thought that the culprit was an infection as well, but to be safe he ordered a CT scan and another round of antibiotics.

That was two weeks ago, and the pain is still there and so is the lump. I haven't heard from the doctor about what the scan showed. That is actually good news, I think. But, on the other hand, it is stressful waiting to hear from him. The main reason is my fear of a recurrence—this is not an irrational fear.

What worries me the most is how a recurrence of cancer for me would affect Susan. Because I follow the same diet that she does, would she lose faith? Would she worry more and stress more and thereby weaken her immune system and . . . ? Well, you get the picture.

I'm not that worried about me because I know I can fight whatever I need to, but I have to admit I haven't had a good night's sleep in weeks, and I am afraid, and I can feel the stress grow by the day.

What a way to start the new year.

Quick Update: Scan Results
By Jeff Weaver — Jan 5, 2014, 9:51 a.m.
Susan and I both got the results of our CT scans on Friday. The good news for Susan was everything looked normal. The problem with her eyes is most likely a side effect of the treatments.

This is a big relief. Her treatments won't change.

But I'm not happy with the message I got from my surgeon. First, it took two weeks and I had to send a request for the results. The email response was composed of two small sentences, each containing fewer than five words. One message said "no further treatment needed." Call me crazy, but I'm a little confused and I would like some clarity.

My lymph nodes are still enlarged, and the antibiotics have not helped. The pain is still there and now has moved to the nodes in the other side of my neck. This could very well be nothing, or it could be something significant.

It seems that because there was no evidence of tumors in my head or neck the doctor thinks there must not be a problem. That doesn't make sense to me. There has to be a reason my nodes are enlarged. I would like to know what that is.

Susan isn't very happy; she insists that I go see my regular doctor and demand we get to the bottom of this. She is going with me to make sure all the questions get asked. You see, I sometimes don't push hard enough. For some reason I don't want to be a pain-in-the-butt patient.

I'll give it some time to make sure the latest round of antibiotics have had a chance to work.

And for Susan, she still has that blood test to see where her estrogen production is. If everything is good, then maybe she can stop the Lupron treatments.

Big Day . . . Sort Of
By Jeff Weaver — Jan 22, 2014, 8:59 a.m.
I think I am more excited about today than Susan is.

Why? For a few reasons. First, Susan turns fifty today! She is not all that happy about it. Must be a woman thing, right? But to me, her turning fifty is a big deal in light of the fact that it is increasingly likely she will see sixty and maybe seventy, and then. . . .

With her CA 27-29 markers still at 32, Susan is defying the odds. But that doesn't surprise me because of everything she does to help increase her odds.

The second reason I'm excited about today is that classes start for me. I finally got the class I need to graduate (Oceanography). So, this spring I will, hopefully, accomplish half of my goal in finishing my education. My goals have changed from when I first started. I wanted to get my master's in economics, but now I want to pursue two other majors, one in creative writing and the other in nutrition and diet. I will start on those this term.

I figured nutrition classes would serve me well if Susan and I end up doing the project we've talked seriously about doing.

I'm the luckiest man alive to have a wife who allows me to pursue my dreams and who is such an inspirational example for me to follow.

Happy birthday, baby. I know the next ten years are going to be awesome. I love you.

Two Years and Counting
By Jeff Weaver — Feb 25, 2014, 3:51 p.m.
As I said, it's been two years since Susan was diagnosed.

A few nights ago I asked Susan what the biggest difference was from year one to year two. Without hesitation she answered, "Work,

work, work." That's it. I just left it at that and didn't ask anything else. As I thought about what she said, it occurred to me that she, unknowingly, might have given me the perfect answer.

Think about what she said for a minute: work, work, work.

Susan is now far more concerned with her job because Macy's is downsizing their workforce and that means smaller crews and more work for her. She's afraid of getting caught up in the downsizing, too. She had to take last week off because she was exhausted from the cumulative effects of her treatments, and her crew is short-handed, so she is working harder. Susan and I have both been around long enough to know that companies look for reasons for who gets to keep their jobs and who gets laid off.

Everyday tasks are now much harder, and to her they feel like work. She is so tired by the time she gets home from Macy's that she doesn't want to cook or do chores around the house, but she does because she is Susan. She is tired from the effects her treatments have on her, so everything she does feels like work.

It's a lot of work to maintain our new lifestyle. We cook from scratch, and that takes time. We have to think about everything we put into her body and what effects the foods have on her. We try to do thirty to forty minutes of exercise every day. We spend lots of time keeping up on research on food and new drugs and treatment options. We understand that we are responsible for her health, and that, my friends, takes work.

Those things are much different from the first year when she worried every day about living or dying.

Speaking of work, in my nutrition class we deal with food and disease. One of my homework assignments was about the cost of obesity in the United States, which is approximately $344 billion a year. We broke that figure down into the cost per group of four people (think families of four) per week. The number turns out to be $88.22. Then we had to figure out what quantity of fruits, veggies, and whole grains (including legumes) we could buy with the $88.22. I was able to buy enough food to feed a four-person group all of the daily recommended servings in each food group and to ensure my "family" got enough of each macronutrient, protein, carbs, and fats. My cost was $87.69.

It's interesting to listen to the twenty-year-olds in class when we talk about eating a healthy diet. They still think they are bullet-proof. They don't understand what the real cost of an unhealthy diet will be.

I'm doing a paper on that. Let me share a few statistics with you.

- One in every three deaths in this country is attributable to poor nutrition and lack of physical activity.
- Sixty-six percent of Americans are overweight; 27 percent of us are obese.
- Thirteen types of cancer are linked to obesity.
- There will be 13 million new cases of cancer worldwide next year, and more than 8 million people die at a cost of $290 billion. In fifteen years, that cost goes up to $458 billion.
- In the United States, 44 percent of men develop cancer, and 23 percent will die.
- Thirty-eight percent of women will get cancer, and 19 percent of them will die.
- In the United States, one in every four deaths is from cancer.
- Of the 3.66 million new cancer cases in the United States next year, 30 percent will be related to obesity and poor nutrition; 96 percent of those are preventable. (Statistics from Centers for Disease Control and Prevention and American Cancer Society)

Those numbers are eye popping, yet we Americans aren't giving up our habits. It takes work to change to a healthy lifestyle. Far too many people want the government to take care of them. . . . It won't. They think that the magic pill is coming to save them. . . . It might, but at what cost? They don't believe the statistics or the science. . . . That's just foolishness. Or they just don't want to change or give up all the "good stuff." . . . That's the hard one.

Susan and I will continue to work on our diet and anything else that we have to do. One thing we have done is back off the rhetoric a little when we talk to people about diet. A couple weeks ago I met my good friend, Peter Gerrard, for coffee. He told me an old joke: How can you tell if a person is a vegan? Just wait a couple minutes and they will tell you. Not sure if he was trying to tell me something, but I do know what he was saying. And I don't want to be that person; I want to be someone who gets things done that will affect the lives of people.

Different Kinds of Victories
By Jeff Weaver — Mar 18, 2014, 12:51 p.m.

When can a cancer patient claim victory in the fight against this deadly disease?

Sometimes it is an easy call, sometimes not so much.

This week I got a message from one of my former writing professors, Shaina Trapedo. In her message she told me about the fourteen-year-old daughter of one of her friends who posted the message "CANCER FREE" on her Facebook page.

This young girl battled cancer and won. She was able to proudly proclaim victory. I don't know the details of her cancer or her fight. But I know I was touched by the message, and I was very proud of that young lady. I told Susan, and she felt the same way.

I sent Shaina a message and asked her to pass along our prayers. I also told her that one of the unique things about cancer is that, for those of us who have fought it or who are fighting it, it's like we are in a special club and we openly root for each other. Consequently, every victory becomes a personal victory for each of us.

I don't even know this girl's name, but it doesn't matter. I know her character and her spirit. I admire her. And I hope she never has to fight this fight again.

Yesterday I was in the cafeteria at school when I got a call from Craig Jackson. Craig and I worked together in Roseburg, Oregon. I knew something was wrong when I heard his voice.

He told me that his wife, Tony, had passed last Thursday. Tony had been in a fierce battle with stage 4 breast cancer for the past five years.

I had talked to her about a year ago. She told me how hard it was to get through each day. She told me about the struggles she had from the get-go. I won't go into the details here, but she wrote an excellent piece that was published in the *News Review* several years ago. The bottom line was, when she was finally diagnosed, she was told she had just a few months to live.

But Tony lived five years longer than anyone thought she was going to. Tony was a tough fighter who didn't give up.

I remember when Craig and Tony first met. I knew they were right for each other. Over time it was apparent how much they loved each other. So, when Craig told me this sad news, I knew how hard this must be for him. But as we talked I could also hear how proud Craig was of her.

Here's the thing: even though cancer took her from him far too soon, Tony did beat the odds. She didn't just fight cancer; in her own way she was victorious.

Tony Jackson is now at peace, and the fight is over. The rest of us can take note of her courage and spirit.

With all the new groundbreaking treatments that target only cancer cells using new and exciting drugs that have been developed or are in trials, the longer those who are fighting cancer can hold out, and thereby increase the chance they might hear, "We can cure you."

Next week Susan has her three-month checkup. So far, she is doing much better than anyone thought was possible. I know she will never give up. After all, she is in a very special club, whose ranks are filled with fighters.

So, here's to victory.

This Is Huge
By Jeff Weaver — Mar 18, 2014, 2:10 p.m.
Okay, so I was wrong. I said Susan's checkup was next week. Nope, it was this morning. And I wasn't there because she didn't remind me this morning, and she couldn't reach me on my cell because I had turned it off last night and forgot to turn it back on.

So, she went alone, and I missed the biggest moment of her two-year fight.

She sent me a text. Her markers are now 30.8. That's down again from three months ago. And the huge part:

Dr. Kashani said . . . wait for it . . .

"YOU ARE IN REMISSION"!!!

Brick Walls
By Jeff Weaver — Jun 15, 2014, 1:05 p.m.

This year Susan and I both crashed through brick walls.

First, let me explain the brick wall thing. A couple Fridays ago, under the fading afternoon sun and the cool breezes that blew in from the beautiful Southern California ocean, I listened to a moving speech by Scott Lay. He is a researcher in constitutional law and international economic and legal systems development at UC Davis's Martin Luther King Hall School of Law. And he has been named one of the top 100 influencers in California politics. These are just a couple of his accomplishments. Scott also was a high school dropout who took a harder road to where he is today.

Scott's speech was about breaking through brick walls. As he put it, brick walls are barriers that less motivated people can't or won't crash through. He said that brick walls are major impediments to life's goals, not mere hurdles, but obstacles that require great energy, planning, drive, determination, and a force of will to get through.

The occasion was my commencement ceremony.

I finally finished phase one of my lifelong pursuit of an education. The latest episode started in the spring of 2009 when I decided to pursue my degree in economics so I could go teach. Turns out it was much more complicated than I thought because nearly all of my old college classes didn't meet the criteria for today's standards. So, I had to retake many of the classes. That was a hurdle on the way to my wall. Other hurdles were my age, which seems to come with a severe memory issue, carving out enough time for my studies because I work so many hours, and, of course the biggest hurdle, Susan's cancer diagnosis. All these hurdles and more were in front of my wall.

How did I break through my brick wall? I watched Susan and marveled at her willingness to do everything she could to fight back against her deadly disease. I thought that if she can sacrifice so much and work so hard, then so can I. I forced myself to study for hours and hours every day, often well into the night. And then I got up at five in the morning when Susan went to work and studied some more. At times I wondered if it was worth the work and stress. But I knew I couldn't give up because I couldn't have Susan see me quit while I asked her to fight on.

As I walked across the stage to receive my diploma, I realized I had broken through my wall, and as I headed back to my seat, I looked around the audience to find Susan (she was the one standing on her chair screaming and yelling), and right behind her I saw another wall. This one is a bigger wall. Behind that wall is a degree in nutrition.

My walls are minor compared to Susan's.

I hope I can frame this so all of you understand how astonishing it is that Susan was able to even make it to her wall. As I think about this, Susan didn't have a wall, she had a nearly impossible barrier in front of her that very few in her position conquer, and the stakes weren't a trophy or a diploma; her life was at stake.

I will never forget the day Susan was told she had cancer or the day we found out she had two separate cancers or the day we found out that both had metastasized. And the worse day ever, when Dr. Asuncion told me that cancer was going to end Susan's life.

That, my friends, is one hell of a big wall.

However, when Susan was first diagnosed we didn't know how big her wall was because the hard part of the fight hadn't started. We had to focus on all of the small barriers in her path. Things like infections, powerful chemo treatments, being unable to work, our ability to pay bills and buy food and cover health insurance premiums.

But I think the biggest challenge we had was when we decided to take matters in our own hands and make wholesale lifestyle changes. The hardest was the dietary changes. For one thing, I didn't know anything about diet and the relationship of food to cancer. Back then we had lots of old bad habits and ate foods that have addictive qualities. It took hundreds of hours to research what not to eat and what to eat in order to give Susan the best chance of beating cancer.

Let me put this in perspective if I can. Every day I talk to people who tell me that someone very close to them has cancer. And at least two times a month I get a call or an email from someone who has cancer asking for help and information. When I tell them what we have done, the answer is usually the same: "Oh, I can't do that" or "I don't want to give up my sweets."

I'm always amazed that folks who are in a fight for their very lives are unwilling to do everything they can to live.

Walls. They are there to keep the weak, the lazy, and the unmotivated out. They aren't usually put up to keep people in.

A few weeks back I was talking to one of my dear friends, Nick Counts, someone I admire and view as a mentor, who told me how much he admired what Susan has done. He said he didn't think people understood just how hard it is to do what she has done. He's right.

Susan is as determined as anyone I've ever met. She is tough, and she is disciplined, and she has the will and strength to do everything she has to do to break through her walls. And as you all know, she broke through her biggest wall when she was told she is in remission.

But, like me when I broke through mine and saw a new wall, so too has Susan.

Yesterday we got a notification that the young navy lieutenant Drew Hilliard just found out that after two years of being clear the cancer is back and it appears to be back in multiple locations. That freaked Susan out.

She said to me, "If his is back, then what's to keep mine from returning, and what's the point of doing what I'm doing?" These were rhetorical questions, of course. But what she was really seeing was her new wall.

Anyone who has taken on a task that is long and difficult to accomplish knows that they have to fight the urges to quit. Some things are a grind, and only grinders will be successful.

Susan's new wall is staying cancer free for five years. She can do that by staying the course with her treatments and her diet. Fighting the urges to take the easy way and resisting the treats people offer her, watching her weight and her attitude, and managing work and home life and her very real fears of recurrence. She must stay focused.

I think it is important for people to understand that being in remission is not the same as being cured. Remission just means the cancer is inactive, but it is still inside a person, working and learning and waiting to fire up in a new more virulent form. Life for Susan will continue to be about living with and fighting cancer. She has no choice in this. I know she dreams of the days when cancer is nothing but a memory.

But for now and the foreseeable future she has to jump whatever hurdles are on her road to a complete victory over cancer.

Dr. Kashani and Susan
By Jeff Weaver — Jun 26, 2014, 8:53 a.m.

Yesterday Susan and I met with Dr. Kashani for her checkup. Her appointment was for 9:50, but we had to wait for over an hour before we were called in. It was much busier than usual in the oncology ward. As we waited I looked around the room at the other patients. Most were older, but there were others Susan's age or younger.

It is easy for me to tell where others are in the treatment cycle. I notice how long their hair is, how thin it is, how gray or faded, often hidden by hats and scarves. Sometimes nervous ticks reveal the stress they are under. Some sit there with their eyes closed. Many of them hold hands with their husbands or wives.

Most of us sitting in oncology waiting rooms find ways to distract ourselves. And I think our anxiety levels are influenced by how advanced the patient's cancer is and how many times we have been in the waiting room—the first couple visits are the most stressful.

All I know for sure is Susan and I have been in those waiting rooms on and off for many years, and the hardest part is the uncertainty of whether the doctor has good news or bad news.

Susan reads and holds my hand. I pass the time by watching others. I try to imagine what they are going through. I worry for them. Often I want to go talk to them. You see, these days, knowing what I know about cancer and lifestyle and diet, I feel the need to help. One thing so many of the cancer patients I see have in common is . . . they are overweight or obese. I can't help wondering if anyone has talked to them about how vital it is to eat correctly, to lose weight, and to exercise so that they have the best chance of beating their disease.

It's hard for me to see these folks, who in many cases are in a desperate fight for their lives, willingly subjecting themselves to harsh and toxic life-shortening drugs and not doing everything they can to increase their survival rates. It's important they take responsibility for their health. They must control what they can and throw everything possible at the disease that is doing everything it can to kill them.

Finally, we were escorted to an exam room. When I sat down in a chair and Susan put on her robe—yup, one of those open-back jobs—I saw a whiteboard on the wall behind her. Written on it in blue and green and black and red was the date, the time, and the doctor's name, plus the name of the nurse who checked the patients in. But what got my attention was the word "survivor" followed by a big red heart and the definition: "To beat the odds, one with great courage & strength, a true inspiration."

I took a picture of the sign because that definition is Susan. In fact, they should put a picture of her next to that sign. Of course, Susan thought I took a picture of her in her air-conditioned hospital gown. She demanded to see my phone, and I gave it to her. Satisfied, she handed it back to me.

When Dr. Kashani came in, he apologized profusely for being so late. He was a little down spirited. He explained that earlier he had to tell one of his patients the worst possible news. He told us that it was a long, tough conversation. I cannot imagine what that must be like.

Then he looked at Susan, and his mood changed from gloomy to bubbly. He told Susan that she looked great and that she was doing great.

For the past couple weeks, Susan has been a real worrywart—especially after reading about Drew Hilliard's recurrence. She has been very tired, which she takes as a sign that something is wrong. So, when Dr. Kashani told her that her CA 27-29 marker was 31.8, it was a relief of sorts. For the first time, her markers had risen since the last visit. Last time they were 30.8. We asked him about the change, and he told us it was normal to see some fluctuation in the numbers. He reminded her that 39 was normal and that she was still far below that number. I'm not sure that helped ease Susan's mind though.

Then we talked a little about the coming changes in health care and how angry he was with it all. And I mean angry. He gets really worked up about this because he won't be able to extend the best care to many of his patients and many of them will have to find another doctor because they are losing their coverage.

Finally, we talked about Susan's treatments going forward. He said, if it ain't broke, don't fix it. I asked how many Aredia treatments she had left; they are the two-hour infusions that fight the cancer in Susan's bones. He said that she would be on them for a long time. The small smile on Susan's face turned to a look of disappointment because the treatments really hurt and the cumulative effects make her joints and bones hurt. She pleaded with him to stop them soon, and he said, "Maybe . . . someday."

As time goes by, her treatments are affecting the quality of her life. All this stuff is toxic and designed to kill cancer cells, but it also is detrimental to healthy cells. He did say he needed to see her only every four months instead of every three months.

That is where we are now. We pray that her markers don't tick up again. I told Susan last night I thought that perhaps because she was taken off the Lupron treatment, the one that suppresses estrogen production, her marker went up a little. It is something we are going to monitor closely. We don't want this thing to blow up on her again.

New CT Scans
By Jeff Weaver — Aug 25, 2014, 10:29 a.m.
For a couple months now Susan has had some discomfort in her lungs and nagging back pain. She emailed Dr. Kashani and he scheduled a CT scan for tomorrow morning.

This is more of a precautionary measure than a real worry. However, the worry on Susan's part is certainly real, and she is genuinely concerned. Ever since Drew Hilliard found out his cancer was back, Susan has been stressing that the same thing will happen to her.

I can't take her mind off it, and I shouldn't promise that she will be okay or that her cancer won't come back, but I do anyway. I remind her how good her doctor is, how hard she fights, and how dedicated she is to lifestyle and diet choices. But I think the best thing that I can do is make sure she knows she isn't alone in this. I let her know how much I love her and how much everyone is pulling and praying for her. I know all these things give her strength.

Susan has been on a much-needed vacation and, boy, did she need the rest. She started a new job at Macy's a few weeks ago as the signing lead. Her old job as the lead merchandiser was very physical, and her treatments had caused the tendons in her wrists to weaken to the point where she could barely lift anything and the pain was excruciating. She had to wear braces that completely immobilized her hands. One of her district managers noticed how much pain she was in and suggested that she take on a new position, one that was less physical and that didn't require much lifting. So, the move was made, and it helped make Susan's life easier. But the added stress of learning a new job isn't good. I know Susan, and she will get this mastered soon. The vacation has given her time to rest and recharge.

I'd like to go back to Susan's constant fear of recurrence. This is a big deal. I know she feels like she has no control over her life at times and that it is only a matter of time before her cancer comes back. The fact is, she has good reason to feel this way. Her doctors told her at the start there was no cure and she had only a few years. I'm sure she hears those words over and over in her mind. I mean, how could she not?

The point I am making here is how much of a burden it is to live like that. Anyone with advanced cancer will tell you that it eats away at your psyche. You can't plan for the future because you can't count on your health holding up. Susan and I can't leave Southern California and go back home to Oregon because we can't afford to lose her insurance or her medical team. And, if we went home, who would give either of us jobs? Because of her cancer and our financial position, one or both of us have to work. All this adds to her sense of helplessness and the feeling of being trapped. When you feel like you have no control over your life, it chips away at your will to fight on as hard as you should.

Metastatic cancer is a thief. It steals energy from your soul. It takes away the everyday joy of living, and it will steal what's left of your life if you are not ever vigilant. Metastatic cancer robs you of the future. I came across a study that hammers home how vigilant cancer patients have to be. The study found that people who have *had* metastatic cancer have a 40 percent chance of recurrence if they have a long-term weight gain of four and a half pounds. Forty percent! And it is especially bad if the weight gain is in the midsection.

Think about that for a second. Who hasn't gained four or five pounds without even noticing it? That's a good thing and a bad thing. Weight gain is harder to control as we age, so we all need to keep a very close eye on the scales. But the good thing about this is it is sort of like the canary in the coal mine: if Susan's weight starts to go up, we can adjust her diet and her exercise program.

One of the most important and telling things, not to mention the most poignant, Susan ever said to me was, "You know, I can't quit. I have to fight as hard as I can because so many people are invested in this fight with me."

Her good friend Cammy Davis sent her a key fob that says: "Just don't give up." I have one, too. It is how we live our lives. Every day I look at those words, and so does Susan.

Scan Results
By Jeff Weaver — Aug 27, 2014, 12:23 p.m.
I just got a call from Susan. She was nearly in tears, so my heart jumped.

She was emotional because the news was great. There are no signs that her cancer has returned. Dr. Kashani was most worried about the pain she was experiencing in her lower spine because the most dangerous part of her cancer had spread to her bones and the biggest concentration was in the pelvic area. Her lungs are clear, too.

This is a huge relief. Susan has been worried sick for weeks now, and this gives her peace of mind for a time.

God, how I hate this disease.

Life Is a Series of Trade-offs and Choices
By Jeff Weaver — Sep 29, 2014, 3:06 p.m.
Yesterday Susan and I participated in the Susan G. Komen Race for the Cure in Newport Beach. I have to say, if you want to support a good cause and go for a 3.2-mile walk with thousands of people, Newport Beach is the place to do it. It was a spectacular day.

We went on the 7:15 a.m. walk. The sun was just rising, the temperature was seventy, the sky was blue, and our spirits were high. This year we went as part of Team Macy's. They had a nice turnout, maybe thirty or so people. Susan got to see a couple of her old friends and managers, Karen and Maria.

This year held a different vibe for us. The first time we did the walk, our daughter, Nicole, organized everything and put together Team Susan. Susan had just finished her harsh round of chemo and was coming off her surgery. Her markers were still high, and her prognosis was grim. Yesterday we were walking for others as much as for Susan. The biggest difference was the absence of Nicole and her friends. We sorely missed their enthusiasm and energy.

As we neared the finish of the race, I saw two groups of protesters. One group held up signs that said Komen supports deadly mammograms and a couple other derogatory statements. The group that really ticked me off was more vocal and the most hateful. They held up signs bashing the Komen Foundation, with one moronic sign saying "30 Years and No Cure." Really! Maybe they don't know that there are over two hundred different types of cancer and that each acts differently and reacts to treatments differently. That means there has to be a specific drug and treatment for each cancer type. Plus, I'm reasonably sure they don't know that cancer learns how we fight it and then morphs into a different form, and that new form requires a different drug. That's why there isn't a cure. Not because, as they shouted, the Komen Foundation does not give enough money to researchers.

I couldn't help myself, so I went over to talk to the protesters. I started by asking, with my best smiley face on, what all this was about. Boy oh boy, they took great delight in informing me how terrible the Susan Komen Foundation is, how Susan Komen treated her sister, how the foundation takes all the money, how the foundation doesn't really want to find a cure because it would then be out of business.

I asked them if they were aware of the good the Komen Foundation does, how much money it gives to research, and then I asked if they thought that Komen was responsible for there not being a cure. (See note at the end of this entry.) I was assaulted with derogatory comments, and my intelligence was called into question. Then I asked the big one, "Well, tell me, just how much time have you put into finding a cure? How much money have you ponied up to find a cure, and tell me exactly what have you done personally to help anyone in their fight against cancer?" More insults and of course the "You don't know anything." There were more personal attacks as I tossed their shiny pamphlets at their feet. They were still yelling at me as I hurried back to the walk and to Susan.

As I jogged up the street, I felt strangely good and angry at the same time. I knew Susan wouldn't be pleased with me. But sometimes you just have to stand up for things. I weigh the risk against the rewards and do what I think I need to do.

That brings me to the point of this entry: life is a series of trade-offs and choices.

What is the difference between a trade-off and a choice? Sometimes it's hard to tell because they are similar. For example, you feel a lump in your breast. Do you decide to get a mammogram, knowing that the risk for women who have regular mammograms is a 50 percent chance of getting a false positive, which is frequently followed by an invasive biopsy? Or do you decide to skip the mammogram and trust luck that you don't have a potentially fatal disease? Let's say you are diagnosed with cancer; you then have a bigger decision to make. Your doctors tell you that you need chemotherapy and inform you of all its health risks, which are many, but the treatments will extend your life or in some cases help you beat the disease. Do you agree to chemotherapy? Or do you forgo the chemo because you don't want to lose your hair or go through the sickness that accompanies it or are afraid of the long-term damage that chemo causes? These are all trade-offs. You get something in exchange for something else.

A choice is different. You choose to buy a $170 pair of designer jeans over a $42 pair of Levis. You choose to be an agent for good by getting involved, by putting yourself, your time, and your money on the line, or you choose to look for fault or to lay blame. You choose to be positive about life or to be a hateful, negative person.

I'm sixty-five and I've done some good things and many not-so-good things because of the choices I've made. And like everyone, I've had my share of trade-offs in life. I've seen how some people have the ability to effect positive change in society and how much good these people do. I've also seen how people can bring down someone's career, business, and life with greed or ambition or, worse, just for the fun of it.

You have many choices in life. You will make many trade-offs as you live it.

Who you are as a person and as a human being is, in large part, determined by the trades-offs and the choices you make along the way. So, don't be like those hateful protesters. Go out and do something to help another human. Be a positive force in someone's life. Being part of the problem or being part of the solution is a choice, and it's yours and yours alone.

Go make a difference.

Note: I looked up in reliable sources how much money Komen donates. In Komen's audited financial statements of 2012, the foundation gave over $58 million in grants to more than a hundred research groups, and in the past thirty years, it has given $685 million. Plus, total donations in all forms is nearly $1.5 billion. These numbers are backed up by an investigative piece written in 2012 for Reuters by two journalists, Sharon Begley and Jane Roberts.

Cancer Wears You Out
By Jeff Weaver — Oct 22, 2014, 10:58 a.m.
I know I've said this before, but I'll say it one last time. The thing about cancer is that it wears you out. If you are fighting cancer, it takes over your life, it consumes you, especially if you are doing what Susan is doing, fighting for all your worth and in every way you can.

Family members of a person battling cancer are also consumed to varying degrees. For example, because Josh lives with us, he is reminded of his mom's battle every day. He sees her when she is down mentally and when she hurts, and he sees the daily toll her treatments have taken. And maybe the worst part is he has heard our conversations about the end of life should things take a turn for the worse. Nicki is spared that sort of thing, but I am certain her mom's fight is on her mind a lot because Susan is Nicki's rock and anchor. As for Ann and Marty, I know Susan's cancer has become a big part of their daily lives.

For everyone who has or is fighting cancer, there is a point when they want to move on to something else. Something different, something new, and something that doesn't suck the life out of you day after day. And for those of us who are so close to and so invested in Susan's fight, we long for something that resembles a normal life.

We want to be set free of cancer.

With that in mind, Susan and I have decided this will be the last entry in her journal.

For months Susan has been winning the fight. Yesterday we met with Dr. Kashani, and he told us her markers are lower than ever before, at 28.6. And the best part was her last CT scan showed no signs of cancer anywhere. None! He and Susan discussed her treatments going forward. I know Susan wants to stop them—who wouldn't, right? She is tired of feeling like crap half of the time, and she is tired of her bones aching and her joints hurting. She is tired of the two-and-a-half-hour Aredia infusions and the five-minute-long shots of Faslodex. But they won't stop and they may never stop because her cancer is considered a chronic disease. However, Dr. Kashani thinks that it is safe to extend the time between Susan's treatments in hopes of alleviating some of the side effects. For this we are both grateful, and we are happy she seems to be beating the very long odds she was given. But our enthusiasm is tempered because we know this may be a lifelong fight and there is still the long-term side effects from all her treatments, so in that respect, there isn't much joy.

Susan and I want to thank everyone who has prayed for and rooted for her and who took time to wish her well. I truly believe that fighting cancer and winning require a lot of help, from medical people, from family, from friends. But, as I said at the start, fighting cancer wears you out.

Susan and I can't move on. She will fight on, and I will be at her side doing everything in my power to help. In the end it's going to boil down to who will wear the other out—Susan or the cancer.

My money is on Susan.

Now a word from the boss . . .

Susan says:

Part of me is doing a happy dance right now because I am so glad Jeff has decided to stop writing about me. Several of my friends and family know how hard it has been for me to have everything made public. Jeff and I have had more than several fights over things that have been written, pictures taken, and even his interpretation of my feelings. I know he has meant well, but I am somewhat of a private person, and some of this has been very hard on me.

But, if it wasn't for everyone who has offered prayers, positive thoughts, and encouragement, I don't think I would have survived. One thing I will never forget is when the surgeon who treated me for that bad infection told me he thought I was going to be all right. His words were the first positive thing I had heard and made me feel like I did have a chance.

I also wouldn't know what tremendous and generous friends I have. I am still overwhelmed by everything that has been done for me. All the love that's been shown for me has made me stronger and helped me fight harder. I never knew how much some people cared about me. But now I do, and it has forever changed me to be a better person.

I will continue to do my best by doing whatever it takes to beat my cancer so I don't disappoint anyone. And so I never have to go through chemo again. That stuff sucks!

I try not to lecture people about how important diet is, but I do wish everyone would try to eat a little better. Had I known a long time ago, I would have made some changes. Not drastic ones, but small ones, because every little bit helps. I know some of my friends and family have, and I'm so proud of them because it's HARD.

All of you should try to make one small change once a month. Try the veggie burger at Red Robin with a side of steamed broccoli. It's not bad! Or make a big batch of oatmeal for a week's worth of breakfasts. That's what I do. I add a lot of cinnamon, clove, nutmeg, banana, and blueberries, and then almond milk with vanilla. I heat it up at my morning break when I'm at work. Makes the whole lunchroom smell yummy. Or make a big bowl of Lemony Kale Salad and eat it with a sandwich instead of chips. Also try making a batch of Lemony Minty Lentil soup and freezing some for a quick dinner during the week. Just defrost it on a busy night.

My point is, I wish everyone would eat better and stay healthy so you don't go through what I have gone through. This hasn't been fun because every day I hurt and I worry about what my treatments are going to do to me after a few more years—and cancer is the reason. It's even harder to watch a loved one go through what I have endured. So, start by making baby changes, and Just Don't Give Up.

With All My Love,

Susan

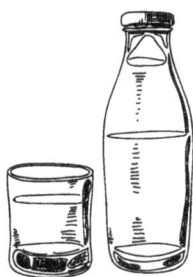

PART II

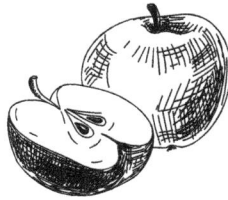

Food Matters

FOR CENTURIES food has been used to help the body perform better physically and mentally, to enhance our mood, to heal wounds, and to cure diseases. Today an enormous amount of scientific evidence proves that eating a plant-based diet helps us live longer and healthier lives. Besides our genes, the foods we eat are the biggest factor in determining the quality and length of our lives.

One thing I would like to make clear is that eating a **moderate amount** of meat and dairy may not harm you. However, people with diabetes, heart disease, and cancer would be well advised to dramatically limit their consumption of most meat and dairy or eliminate these foods altogether. It is easy to consume all the nutrients and protein the body needs from plants. As strong as the science is on how certain foods can help heal us, science has also found that eating certain foods on a regular basis causes chronic health problems that often lead to painful and premature death.

The most common diet-related conditions that are detrimental to our health are chronic inflammation, belly fat, atherosclerosis, and a weakened immune system. All these conditions can be virtually eliminated, or at the very least dramatically reduced, by dietary choices.

Inflammation has long been associated with cancer. It is way too complicated a topic to fully explain here, in part because our bodies use inflammation to help fight diseases, but too much inflammation is harmful. Basically, chronic inflammation leads to the development of dysplasia, which is the enlargement of an organ or tissue by proliferation of cells of abnormal types. Rapid cell growth and out-of-control cell replication occur in the development of cancer. Nearly 15 percent of cancer worldwide is a result of inflammation, according to a study published in the *Yale Journal of Biology and Medicine*.

There are two types of fat in and around our abdomen: subcutaneous fat (the stuff we can grab with our hands) and visceral fat, which is inside the abdominal cavity and which acts as a buffer between the organs located there. According to a paper published in 2012 by Harvard Medical School, when we have an excess of visceral fat—belly fat—we are at a much "higher risk of cardiovascular disease, type 2 diabetes, gallbladder disease and breast cancer." The piece also states that fat cells, especially abdominal fat, are "biologically active and act like an organ or gland by producing hormones and other substances that profoundly affect our health."

Visceral fat also causes insulin resistance, which means the body's muscle and liver cells can no longer adjust to normal levels of insulin, creating much higher levels of glucose in the bloodstream. This excess glucose causes the body to produce too many cells, which often leads to cancer. Plus, too much insulin increases estrogen production, which changes in a way that promotes breast cancer.

Atherosclerosis is a cardiovascular disease caused by the buildup of lipids and scar tissue formed by injury to the cells that line the insides of arteries. This buildup causes a narrowing of the vessels. Common factors that promote vessel injury are blood forcefully pounding against the artery walls (high blood pressure; think of a hose with a nozzle—the narrower the aperture of the nozzle, the more force the water stream has coming out of the hose), damage from irritants in tobacco, and excessive glucose in the blood stream. These all lead to vessel inflammation, which is increasingly recognized as the root cause of cardiovascular disease.

The inflamed vessels allow lipids (fats, oils, and triglycerides) to seep through the layers of the vessel walls into the vessels, where they become trapped and accumulate in deposits known as plaque. As plaque forms, it restricts blood flow to the body's tissues, resulting in the withering of tissues and the loss of their ability to function.

Heart attacks and strokes are the most commonly known cardiovascular diseases. Less well known is the relationship between cancer and atherosclerosis. The development and progression of atherosclerosis and cancer share a series of molecular pathways with a common origin. It has been found that both diseases develop from a clonal proliferation of damaged cells where there is tissue injury, inflammation, and gene instability. This is a very complicated subject and requires more time and space to explain than I have here. The simplified version is: estrogen and androgen hormone production, the development of atherosclerosis, and DNA mutations that result from oxidative stress are associated. Mutated estrogen and androgen genes are the genus of breast, genital tract, and prostate cancers.

Much of this is not yet fully understood, but what is known is the dietary link. Whereas omega-3 fatty acids help protect the body's cells from atherosclerosis and cancer, consumption of large amounts of saturated fats leads to gene mutations and excessive cell proliferation. Overweight people are at a much higher risk.

A bigger problem for cancer patients who also have atherosclerosis is, because the arteries and blood vessels are constricted, the body cannot defend itself against cancer because not enough white bloods cells can get to areas affected by excessive cell proliferation. And their normal cells aren't getting enough vital nutrients to function properly and effectively. These conditions enable cancer cells to proliferate at a high rate and thus consume more and more of the body's fuel, stealing food from the healthy cells. This is really what kills a person: cancer starves the normal cells of the fuel they need to survive.

By eliminating the foods that cause atherosclerosis and by switching to foods that repair the damage done to our cardiovascular system, we can increase the health and efficiency of the immune system and increase blood flow, which supplies vital nutrients and oxygen to healthy cells.

The blood vessels that feed normal cells differ from the networks of blood vessels that cancer creates to feed cancerous cells. New research shows that certain foods may suppress the creation of these malignant blood vessel networks. It is also known that certain foods prevent cancer cells from absorbing nutrients, thus stopping them from proliferating. Finding out how and why this happens may be an important key in finding a cure for cancer.

The **immune system** is the body's army of natural killers. Its only job is to seek out and kill infections, viruses, and diseases such as cancer. If our immune system weakens, we are more susceptible to diseases and infections and less able to fight them when we are affected by them.

Diet plays a vital role in the health of our immune system. For example, a crash diet of fewer than twelve hundred calories per day can greatly reduce immune function; on the other hand, excessive energy intake via overeating also compromises the immune system's ability to ward off diseases. For most of us, when we take in more calories than we burn, we gain weight, and over time that can lead to obesity. People who are obese have weaker immune systems, which leads to increased rates of infections and higher rates of coronary disease, which further weakens the immune system. On the plus side, many foods help strengthen the immune system, thus enabling the body to better defend itself.

Foods, Spices, and Herbs

All the foods Susan and I eat either directly or indirectly have some cancer-fighting component or property. Our goal is to help her fight and hopefully defeat cancer. I see that she gets all of the essential nutrients, vitamins, and minerals. And to maximize the effectiveness of the food, it matters how the foods in a meal are paired and it matters when certain foods are eaten. Some vitamins and other nutrients are better absorbed when eaten in the right combinations, and the body has different nutritional needs at different times of the day. Do a simple Internet search for pairing foods to maximize health effects and you will find a lot of useful information.

Here are a few important facts to know. Calories matter for all people because if we consume too many calories we **will gain weight** regardless of the claims made in favor of different types of diets. Awareness of calorie consumption is especially important for cancer patients because research shows that just a four-and-a-half-pound long-term gain in weight results in a 40 percent chance of recurrence. And how much of the three major sources of energy—carbohydrates, proteins, and fats—make up a diet really matters. For example, the energy provided by 1 gram of carbohydrate or 1 gram of protein equals 4 kilocalories (kcals; we call them calories in the United States), whereas 1 gram of fat supplies 9 kcals. This is why you need to be careful with fat intake because fat is very calorie dense; you can't eat the same volume of fat as you do of carbs or proteins.

Carbohydrates are the primary source of fuel for the body. Carbs are what the body uses for physical activities, brain function, and operation of our organs. All cells and tissues rely on carbs to function.

Proteins have a couple different functions in the body. Their main role is to act as a structural component of cells and tissue. Protein helps repair damaged tissue and serves as a source of fuel if enough carbohydrates or fats are unavailable.

Fat is a concentrated source of energy and is essential because it is the body's first source of fuel when carbs aren't available. This is why the body stores fat rather than uses it right away. The dietary fats we consume are the major fuel source for our body while at rest. Around 30 to 70 percent of the energy our muscles and organs use when we are inactive comes from the fats we have eaten. Plus, only fats can absorb the essential vitamins A, D, E, and K.

So, how do you decide how much of each macronutrient group to eat when trying to figure out what is right for you? Each person has different energy needs depending on activity and body weight as well as overall health. Susan is at 1,800 calories or fewer a day, with

65 percent coming from carbohydrates, 20 percent from protein, and 15 percent from fats. If this calculation is not something you can do on your own, consult with a registered dietitian—not your doctor, unless he or she is trained in nutrition. Just a side note here: after Susan was diagnosed with cancer and we knew diet could be a key component in her fight, we decided to change our family doctor to one who uses food and lifestyle as integral parts of patient care. Nowadays food as medicine is seeing a revival of sorts, and more and more doctors are revisiting the idea of using food as a treatment option.

Planning a diet in this way takes a lot of work and is hard to do. One thing that helps us stay on track is a free phone app that tracks this information and that is supereasy to use. The app, MyFitnessPal, allows you to set goals for carbs, fat, protein, and calories. It also has a barcode reader that makes it easy to input foods by hand. It includes a wide variety of foods in its database. It shows us most of the nutritional content of the foods we consume. I think it was a key factor in our success.

What I found out quickly is that I had to measure portion sizes to get an accurate reading of calorie and nutrient intake. I can't stress this enough: you have to know what you are putting into your body and how much of it. Once I started using the app, my weight and my waistline started melting away at a steady pace. And you have to be honest when you measure and enter data because, if you want to succeed, you can't cheat. By the way, I have lost 60 pounds and now weigh 172 pounds.

Before I list the foods, spices, and herbs that we use in our diet, I want to say that I did hundreds of hours of research on the subject and went so far as to take college nutrition classes. One important thing I learned was to find out who was behind the study or research and who put up the money. As I said in the introduction, there are a lot of agenda-driven research pieces out there, and I wanted only the most accurate information I could find.

Nearly every study I read came with disclaimers or qualifying words such as "Further studies need to be done" or "may have some cancer-fighting properties." However, those statements are more a cover-your-butt thing than an indication of the uncertainty of the science. So, maybe it's prudent I add my own disclaimer:

Your results may vary.

Basically, most of the food Susan and I eat is made up of whole foods rather than processed; also, it is plant based. However, if so inclined, we could also eat certain foods that aren't plant based, such as sardines, tuna, wild-caught salmon from Alaska, and other wild-caught fish from Alaska. The problem with most fish is that the toxins they ingest or absorb from the highly polluted waters they live in gets passed to us when we eat them. I would never prepare farm-raised fish for Susan because of all the antibiotics and hormones they are given and artificial foods they are fed to accelerate growth.

Other items I try to avoid are genetically modified organisms (GMO) or, in our case, genetically modified foods. Not because I'm politically against genetic modification of foods but because enough scientific evidence warrants erring on the side of caution. Until there is conclusive evidence that GMO foods are completely safe, Susan and I opt for natural foods. We use organic produce because, again, the science is pretty firm that toxic residues of the pesticides and synthetic fertilizers used in commercial farming transfer into the food. We don't use high heat in cooking, which means no frying foods above a medium heat setting. The National Cancer Institute says that frying food creates acrylamide, a known carcinogen, which is a "major concern" when it comes to cancer. We also try to avoid canned tomatoes (this is not always possible) because the cans are lined with bisphenol A (BPA), an epoxy resin used in food packaging. Tomatoes are high in acid, which causes the carcinogenic compound BPA to leach into the tomatoes. While I'm on the subject of BPA, we use only BPA-free water containers to drink from.

Studies have shown that many foods, herbs, and spices contain specific vitamins, compounds, and phytochemicals, along with other substances, that are known for their ability to stimulate and aid the body's immune system and, thus, help prevent cancer. In some instances, these substances may even aid in the reversal of certain types of cancer.

Let's start with foods we use as main ingredients.

Legumes: Dry Beans, Split Peas, and Lentils

Kidney beans, red and black beans, yellow split peas, red lentils, and, one of my favorites, chickpeas—also called garbanzo beans (technically, these are seeds)—are among the hundreds of colorful legumes. Legumes use nitrogen from the atmosphere to make protein and are an important protein source in plant-based diets. One serving (1 cup) of chickpeas provides a whopping 15 grams of protein, 12 grams of fiber, only 4 grams of fat, and 26 percent of your daily iron requirements. One cup of black beans has about 12 grams of protein and 10 grams of fiber. Legumes are an excellent source of the B vitamin folate. They also contain antioxidants from a variety of phytochemicals such as triterpenoids, flavonoids, inositol, protease inhibitors, and sterols.

Whole Grains

Whole grains such as brown rice, oats, corn, wheat, barley, bulgur, kasha, millet, and farro have fiber-rich bran, nutrient-packed germ, starchy endosperm, and all-natural nutrition and health-promoting phytochemicals, including phenolic acids and flavonoids. They also have known cancer-fighting compounds such as lignins, saponins, phytic acid, as well as protease inhibitors that may stop cancer from spreading.

Whole grains are good sources of fiber and protein. Some, like corn, are high in resistant starch, which is a unique starch that resists digestion and which aids in weight loss, increases the body's ability to burn fat, helps control blood sugar levels, and boosts the immune system. Whole grains are also good sources of manganese, thiamine, niacin, vitamin B6, and selenium.

Seeds

Seeds pack a big health punch for their size. They are high in protein, fiber, iron, calcium, magnesium, and omega-3 fatty acids. For example, a little-known powerhouse is hemp seed. Three tablespoons of hemp seed provide 10 grams of complete protein, 15 percent of our daily iron needs, and both omega-3 and omega-6 fatty acids. One of our go-to seeds is quinoa because it is interchangeable with rice and it has 6 grams of protein per serving. About 4 tablespoons of ground flaxseed, one serving, contains more than 7 grams of fiber, and about half of the fat in flaxseed is a form of omega-3 fat and is high in vitamin E.

Other really healthful and great-tasting seeds are chia, cumin, pomegranate, and pumpkin.

Dark Leafy Greens
Spinach, kale, romaine lettuce, leaf lettuce, mustard greens, collard greens, chicory, Swiss chard, and arugula (which is also called garden rocket) are excellent sources of fiber, folate, and a wide range of carotenoids such as lutein, zeaxanthin, saponins, and flavonoids.

Studies show that foods containing carotenoids likely protect against cancer. Carotenoids seem to prevent cancer by acting as antioxidants and then scouring dangerous free radicals from the body before they can do harm. Research has also found that the carotenoids in dark green leafy vegetables can inhibit the growth of certain types of breast cancer, skin cancer, lung cancer, and stomach cancer cells.

Lately, a few articles tell us we shouldn't eat kale because too much might harm us by causing hypothyroidism. What those articles don't say is that we would have to eat 3 pounds 5 ounces a day for several months to do the body harm. So, weigh that risk against the benefits of eating just one serving, which is 1 cup or 2.36 ounces, daily. Along with the above-mentioned benefits, the indoles and nitrogen compounds in kale help stop lesions from turning into cancerous cells in estrogen-sensitive tissue that are found in breasts, ovaries, colons, and prostates. Also, kale is rich in isothiocyanate and phytochemicals that help stop tumors from growing and keep cancer-causing substances from even reaching our cells.

Dark leafy greens should make up a significant part of your diet. We grow all our kale, Swiss chard, and watercress in a small garden because they are easy to grow, don't require a lot of space, and are pesticide-free. They also grow well in medium- to large-sized containers and pots.

Cruciferous Vegetables
Cruciferous vegetables are some of the best cancer-fighting foods around. They are household names yet often ignored or not included in our meals because of their distinctive flavor. Cruciferous vegetables include broccoli, brussels sprouts, rapini, cabbage, cauliflower, radishes, and turnips (white). Others, known as "headless crucifers," are dark green leafy vegetables such as arugula, kale, and collards.

These all are excellent or good sources of vitamin C, and some are good sources of manganese. Dark greens are high in vitamin K and fiber and rich in magnesium. The cancer-fighting compounds glucosinolates, which form isothiocyanate and indole, are found in all cruciferous vegetables along with other nutrients, phytochemicals, and vitamins, including folate (a B vitamin) and potassium. Plus, they contain carotenoids such as beta-carotene and supply anthocyanins along with polyphenols, such as hydroxycinnamic acids, kaempferol, and quercetin, all of which are known for their anticancer effects. These compounds not only slow down the growth of cancer cells but also help shrink tumors in some cases.

Studies suggest that cruciferous vegetables protect the body from most types of cancer, including bladder, colorectal, stomach, prostate, and lung cancers. This is especially true of all cabbages. Cabbage, especially Savoy cabbage, is a great source of sinigrin. Sinigrin, a glucosinolate, converts into allyl-isothiocyanate, a compound that research shows has a unique cancer-preventing property with respect to bladder, colon, and prostate cancers.

This group makes up a very large part of Susan's diet. Research has shown that women with breast cancer who eat more cruciferous vegetables have a 62 percent higher survival rate and 35 percent reduction in recurrence. This is, in part, because foods such as kale, broccoli, cabbage, and cauliflower contain indole-3-carbinol, which helps fight breast cancer by converting cancer-promoting estrogen to a type of estrogen that does not promote breast cancer. We find ways to include crucifers in a wide variety of dishes and eat them as standalone dishes.

Nuts

All nuts include antioxidants, which help protect your body from the cellular damage that contributes to heart disease, cancer, and premature aging, and they, especially walnuts, fight inflammation. Nuts also help lower cholesterol levels and heart disease risk and can aid in weight control if eaten judiciously (because they are calorie dense). Nuts are high in fiber and good sources of protein, iron, zinc, vitamin E, and calcium. A one-ounce serving of Brazil nuts, about six nuts, have 100 percent of the daily amount of selenium, which is a known cancer fighter.

University of Texas MD Anderson Cancer Center researchers found that eating two ounces of pistachios daily may reduce lung cancer risk. Pistachios are rich in the antioxidant gamma-tocopherol, a form of cancer-fighting vitamin E. Pistachios are also packed with potassium. Of the nuts, almonds contain the most vitamin E, which is a powerful antioxidant.

New research just published in the *International Journal of Epidemiology* found that people who ate tree nuts such as almonds, cashews, and walnuts and peanuts (not a tree nut) reduced their risk of dying from cancer, heart disease, and respiratory illness and the incidence of neurodegenerative diseases, such as Alzheimer's and Parkinson's. It's best to eat raw nuts rather than roasted and salted nuts.

Herbs and Spices

Some of the best cancer fighters are in this group. Herbs and spices can easily be added to any dish, not only to enhance the flavors but also to enhance the cancer-fighting ability of the dish. Scientists have found that phytochemicals in many herbs and spices can affect our bodies at a biological level because of their ability to stimulate the immune system. The stronger our immune system is, the better equipped our bodies are at fighting off infections and diseases, including cancer. Use as many and as much spices and herbs as you can.

Turmeric, one of the best cancer fighters, contains curcumin, which gives turmeric its yellow color. Curcumin is one of the most powerful anti-inflammatories ever identified. Cancer tumors have a network of blood vessels that feed them, and curcumin can work against these blood vessels and essentially choke off the blood flow to cancer cells, thus depriving them of the glucose they require to grow and propagate.

Garlic, along with onions, shallots, scallions, and leeks, are allium vegetables that may help prevent cancer, especially of the stomach. Allium vegetables contain organosulfur compounds that strengthen the immune system because of their powerful anti-inflammatory properties and they have anticarcinogenic qualities. These foods may be vegetables, but we use them to spice up dishes.

Fresh ginger has been used as medicine for thousands of years. It is in the same family as turmeric and cardamom. It's known for its ability to control and relieve nausea and vomiting from several causes, among them chemotherapy. Some of the other things ginger does is help stimulate circulation, inhibit rhinovirus (which causes common colds), and inhibit bacteria such as *Salmonella*. Ginger is one of the most effective anti-inflammatories out there. Fresh ginger contains gingerol and, when dried, forms zingerone. Both have antioxidant and anti-inflammatory properties and therefore help protect against cancer.

Hot peppers in any form—fresh, flaked, and ground—are one of our go-to spices because they are high in antioxidants and anti-inflammatory properties, giving hot peppers their superior cancer-fighting abilities. The compound capsaicin is found in all hot peppers. Capsaicin is so powerful that laboratory studies show that it can induce apoptosis, or programmed cell death, in up to 80 percent of active prostate cancer cells, or, in other words, it induces cancer cell suicide. Other studies show hot chili peppers are effective at fighting several types of cancer, including breast cancer, and other types of inflammation-driven diseases.

Oregano is a superspice. It contains vitamins A, C, E, B6, and K plus has fiber, folate, iron, magnesium, calcium, and potassium. It has anti-inflammatory properties along with antimicrobial effects. Research shows it may kill MRSA, *Listeria*, and other pathogens. Biologists at the United Arab Emirates University reported that oregano "exhibits anticancer activity by encouraging cell cycle arrest and apoptosis [cell death] of the MDA-MB-231 breast cancer line." Plus, they think it will "slow or prevent the progression of cancer in patients with breast cancer."

Black pepper contains the active substance piperine, a naturally occurring chemical compound with strong antioxidant properties. A study conducted by scientists at the University of Michigan Comprehensive Cancer Center and published in the journal *Breast Cancer Research and Treatment* found pepper along with turmeric inhibited the growth of cancerous stem cells of breast tumors.

I spend a lot of time trying to figure out how to incorporate herbs and spices into my dishes. It's where I get the flavor that amps up my recipes and makes my food very potent cancer-combatting meals.

Fruits and Berries

Fruits are by design a nearly perfect food. Because human bodies don't produce vitamin C, we must obtain it from the foods we eat. Fruits are the best source of vitamin C, which is essential for maintaining health and even life. Our bodies also need to constantly resupply many of the key vitamins and phytocompounds that are abundant in fruit. Eating a lot of fruit helps build bone density, and fruits have other well-known disease-fighting capabilities.

Fruits are full of cancer-fighting and anti-inflammatory

compounds. For example, pineapples contain the enzyme bromelain, which is a known cancer fighter. Cherries have the compound anthocyanin, which has been shown to effectively reduce pain and inflammation. Pomegranates contain potent plant estrogens that do not stimulate unregulated cell proliferation and that are packed with anti-inflammatory compounds. Red grapes have the potent antioxidant resveratrol, which, among other things, helps prevent the onset of Alzheimer's, helps repair cells by protecting against free radicals, and is known to prevent the growth of cancer cells. Elderberries are high in flavonoids, which compare favorably with the antiviral drug Tamiflu at binding to and preventing H1N1 infection.

Tomatoes are really a fruit and have many bioactive compounds such as vitamins E and C, polyphenols, and carotenoids such as lutein and lycopene. Research suggests that they inhibit tissue-damaging compounds, and they have been found to lower the risk of several cancers and help reduce cardiovascular disease. Watermelon actually has 40 percent more of the cancer fighter lycopene than do tomatoes along with high levels of vitamins A, C, B6, thiamine, and potassium.

Apples are on the "dirty dozen" list every year because of the pesticides used by commercial growers, so I recommend buying organic apples whenever possible. That said, apples are a powerful health food. They have been shown to reduce the risk of cancer because they are high in fiber, phytochemicals, and flavonoids, such as quercetin, myricetin, kaempferol, and catechin. Plus, apples are the highest in phenolic antioxidants (PAs), which are found only in plants. These types of antioxidants help protect us from arthritis, cancer, and other inflammation-driven diseases by preventing tissue inflammation and from DNA damage at the cellular level. PAs also reduce the oxidation that causes cells to die and that helps cancer tumors grow.

One of the best sources of vitamin C is papaya. Papaya is also high in beta-carotene as well as other carotenoids, plus it has plenty of vitamin E—all of which make this fruit a top resource for fighting inflammation. And I think it tastes wonderful, not like dirt as Susan thinks.

Susan eats mango nearly every day because she loves it and it is high in vitamins C, A, B6, and K, folate, and potassium. Mangoes are high in fiber along with the antioxidants beta-carotene and zeaxanthin. They help decrease the risk of macular degeneration and colon cancer, improve digestion, and help strengthen bones. She supercharges them by adding fresh minced ginger root, chili powder, a little lime, and sliced strawberries.

Fruits, especially citrus, are a mainstay in our kitchen because they are packed with nutrition and are essential for delivering the flavors that make our food so good. Plus, there is such a wide variety of fruits, and some are always in season, which means they taste better and are higher in nutritional value.

Berries are good sources of vitamin C and fiber. Studies show foods high in vitamin C help protect against cancer of the esophagus and foods containing dietary fiber decrease the risk of colorectal cancer.

All berries, particularly strawberries and black and red raspberries, are rich in ellagic acid. In laboratory studies, this phytochemical was shown to prevent cancers of the skin, bladder, lung, esophagus, and breast. Research suggests that ellagic acid seems to utilize several different cancer-fighting methods at once because it acts as an antioxidant and it helps the body deactivate specific carcinogens, plus it helps slow the reproduction of cancer cells.

Strawberries also contain a wide range of other phytochemicals called flavonoids, which seem to fight cancer in a variety of ways. Blueberries contain a family of phenolic compounds called anthocyanosides, which many scientists believe are among the most potent antioxidants yet discovered.

The bottom line is, berries of all sorts are powerful weapons against cancer. New studies have found that when different types of berries are combined their cancer-fighting properties are strengthened.

We use berries in everything, from toppings on cereals to salads, from flavoring main dishes to—of course—adding to smoothies and serving as evening snacks.

Mushrooms

Mushrooms are fungi. They are also one of the top foods in our diet because of their ability to reduce the risk of cancer. Many studies show they may even help reverse cancer. Mushrooms have been a mainstay in medicine for centuries. Mushrooms are high in glycoproteins and polysaccharides, which assist cell communication. This enables hormones, chemical messengers, to be more efficient by making sure cells get the appropriate messages faster. This is important because more precise messaging helps the immune system distinguish between rogue cells and healthy cells more quickly. The body's defense system can then target and attack mutant cells.

Mushrooms have other potent immune system agents in them, such as funnel proteins, lectins, and peptides.

Research suggests that eating mushrooms helps increase survival time for cancer patients and helps mitigate the side effects of chemotherapy and radiation treatments. Some science even suggests mushrooms may help shrink cancer tumors; however, more studies need to be done.

The best ones are maitake, shiitake, cordyceps, reishi, and portobello. Mushrooms are a powerful food in the fight against cancer.

Green Tea and African Red Tea

Green tea should be a big part of your diet. It's hard to read any health-related piece without running across the virtues of green tea. One thing you don't see too often is the qualifier that decaffeinated green tea is a better choice. That is because it is richer in catechin, an antioxidant that plays a major role in cancer prevention. Laboratory studies show that catechin slows or prevents the development of cancer in the colon, liver, breast, esophageal, and prostate cells. It also contains the chemicals EGCG and ECG, which are free-radical-fighting compounds that prevent DNA damage.

Another benefit of green tea, because of its high levels of polyphenols and antioxidants, is that it helps repair sun damage to the skin from exposure to damaging UV rays that often results in skin cancers. It also helps fight depression because of the amino acids it contains.

African red tea, also called rooibos tea, has been found to be higher in antioxidants than other teas. Antioxidants help protect healthy cells from damage by clearing our bodies of free radicals. Free radicals are unstable molecules that attack and steal electrons from surrounding stable molecules in an attempt to gain stability. When a molecule loses an electron, it is converted into a free radical, which is unstable and reacts quickly to steal an electron from a nearby stable molecule. This process cascades until damage occurs at the cellular level. This damage creates inflammation, which, as we know, can lead to many diseases, including cancer.

Red tea is also naturally decaffeinated, which makes it a perfect choice for kids and people who are sensitive to the effects of caffeine.

Other Cancer-Fighting Foods

Two other foods we eat regularly are essential to our dietary war on cancer because they are nutritious, loaded with anticancer compounds, and are versatile. **Avocados** are high in the powerful antioxidant glutathione, which helps destroy free radicals by blocking the intestines from absorbing bad fats. They are believed to help protect against liver cancer. Avocados have more potassium than bananas and are loaded with beta-carotene.

Instead of regular potatoes (we do eat them occasionally), we eat **sweet potatoes** and **red yams** a couple times a week. They are a great source of beta-carotene, which helps protect DNA in our cells. The dark varieties of sweet potatoes have more cancer-fighting carotenoids in them. They are also a good source of potassium and are high in vitamins C and B6, iron, manganese, lutein, zeaxanthin, and copper. No wonder they are on the "Worlds Healthiest Foods" list.

☁

The key to using food as medicine is to do your homework and, if you can, consult a registered dietitian or nutritionist who has experience with diet and disease. Make sure your diet is well balanced so you get all the essential vitamins and nutrients.

Science clearly shows a plant-based diet is best if you have chronic cancer or if you just want to reduce the risk of ever getting cancer, heart disease, and diabetes. I have read many articles about how hard it is to get all the essential nutrients from a plant-based diet. In fact, those against plant-based diets—that is, the meat and dairy industries—most often make that assertion.

However, after I did some studying, I found it wasn't at all hard to eat a totally balanced diet. I would argue that people who eat a whole foods, plant-based diet actually consume more essential nutrients because they have a higher awareness of what they put into their bodies in comparison to people who eat a typical Western diet, who are usually deficient in more nutrient categories. People who eat a standard Western diet are prone to consuming far too much fat and protein at the expense of the best foods nature has to offer: whole grains, vegetables, greens, and fruits.

The other thing I hear constantly is that eating an organic plant-based diet is just too expensive. Truth is, it is actually cheaper to eat this way—not because we eat organic but because we *don't* eat high-cost foods such as meat, cheese, and prepackaged processed foods. When we first went on our diet, we were dead broke and had about $50 to $60 a week to spend on food . . . if that. We got good at shopping for what we really needed and where the best places were to buy it. Plus, I started growing most of our herbs and greens at home. What is costly, in one sense, is the time it takes to plan meals and prepare the food.

Nowadays it's not hard to find information on how foods fight many diseases and help prevent hundreds of health-related problems. Poor food choices are a big reason why Americans suffer from so many disabling and deadly conditions. In my view, this condition is only going to get worse in the coming decades.

Susan and I were walking around the Brea Mall last weekend, and she said to me, "Look at how big people are getting, even the young kids." It's something I have noticed everywhere I go. She didn't say that in a mean-spirited way either; on the contrary, she is saddened because she knows most of these folks don't realize that they are putting themselves at much higher risk of going through what she is.

Medical professionals know for a fact that obesity is one of the big contributing factors to various chronic diseases. So, going forward, America can expect an explosion in the numbers of health problems such as heart disease, diabetes, and cancer. **This will cost us billions of dollars and millions of lives.** What that means is we are mortgaging our future and the future of our kids and grandchildren. But that is a discussion for another day.

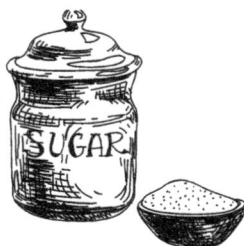

Foods Not to Eat

SOMEONE WHO has ever been diagnosed with cancer should *never* eat anything on this list. I don't list everything that should be avoided here because that would make a very long list made up of additives and chemicals whose names most of us can't even pronounce. However, a handful of common foods top the list.

Sugar

For any cancer patient, processed or refined sugar is the single most important food to never eat. Often referred to as simple sugar, it has many names and forms. In fact, there are over one hundred different names that are on food ingredient lists (Google this and take notes). Also, any carbohydrate that has been refined or processed should be treated as a simple sugar and, therefore, avoided. Think white rice and white bread and other like foods. I have mentioned many times that sugar is the food of choice for cancer. Cancer cells consume up to forty times more glucose than healthy cells. If a cancer patient eats sugar, it's like pouring gas on a fire. That alone is enough to put sugar at the top of the list; however, everyone would be well advised to avoid sugar. Most well-respected food scientists now think sugar is as bad as smoking when it comes to causing chronic health problems. I tell people that if they could do only one thing, cut sugar from their diet . . . today!

Hundreds of studies have been done on the effects of sugar on the human body. In fact, added sugar is now considered the most dangerous ingredient we eat. A new study published in the journal *Obesity* and reported in *Forbes* found that the weight gain associated with sugar consumption is only the tip of the problem. The study found that sugar brought about distinct metabolic changes that have nothing to do with weight gain.

The strictly controlled trial was done on obese children who had a metabolic condition such as high blood pressure, high triglyceride levels, or markers for fatty liver. The researchers reduced the percentage of calories the kids normally consumed through sugar intake by 65 percent. Plus, they made sure the kids' weight did not change by adding back the same number of calories from starches.

After just nine days all the kids experienced significant metabolic changes. Researchers found that every child had lower blood pressure, triglycerides had fallen 33 points, bad LDL cholesterol was down 10 points, insulin levels went down 33 percent, and "fasting glucose and liver functions improved."

Cutting sugar from the diet also means you have to stop eating foods made with refined grains, such as white bread, white rice, and most boxed cereals, because refined grains turn into glucose quickly and flood the bloodstream with excess glucose. You also must learn to read labels to see if sugar has been added.

Alcohol

According to the American Cancer Society and the National Cancer Institute, there are many reasons to stop drinking alcohol if you have cancer. For starters, drinking can have a negative effect on the course of cancer treatments. Then there is the fact that alcohol can irritate the throat and mouth, causing open sores. This can lead to infections because cancer treatments lower the body's white blood cell count, making it harder to combat infections.

For any cancer survivor, consuming alcohol increases the risk of recurrence. It will "reduce nutrients in the blood that are protecting against cancer," thus depriving the body's healthy cells of those nutrients.

Alcohol raises the levels of estrogen in the body, which makes it one of the worst things a breast cancer patient can consume.

Another harmful side effect of drinking alcohol is the very real risk of weight gain, and that is an important consideration because being overweight increases the risk of many types of cancer. Alcohol is known to cause liver damage, which leads to inflammation that ends up damaging our DNA. It also slows the body's ability to "break down and get rid of some harmful chemicals."

Then there are the known effects alcohol has on a person's "mood, concentration, judgement and coordination." When you are fighting cancer, mood and judgment (decision making) are big deals because studies show that people with better moods have higher rates of recovery and that making bad dietary choices has a dramatic effect on the patient's outcome.

Dairy Products

The next two—dairy products and red meat—are the hardest to stop eating and the most defended foods on the list. However, registered dietitians who specialize in diet for cancer patients advise cancer patients, especially those with breast cancer, against eating dairy products.

A study conducted by researchers at Kaiser Permanente found that "women diagnosed with early stage breast cancer who ate full-fat dairy . . . are more likely to die from breast cancer." Estrogen is a hormone created from fat and stored in fat cells. This is important to note because full-fat dairy products are produced mostly by pregnant cows, making their milk much higher in estrogen. The extra estrogen gets stored in a woman's fat cells and eventually causes a rise in their estrogen levels. Estrogen is a known "stimulant for breast cancer growth."

In a follow-up study, Kaiser researchers studied 1,500 of the women who participated in the original study and who had made the switch to low-fat dairy. They followed them for 12 years. They found that 349 women had suffered a recurrence and 189 had died "specifically from breast cancer." These recurrence and death rates are still high when compared to the rates of women who limit consumption of dairy products, so it's not just the fat content alone that is dangerous. The question then is, is there something else in dairy that causes the added cancer risk?

One link to cancer exists in the two cancer-prone glands: prostate and breast. The link is the 5alpha-pregnane-dione (5a-P) that is found in milk. The steroid 5a-P has been found to be a direct pathway in prostate cancer. Additionally, 5a-P is capable of bringing about estrogen receptors for breast cancer cells that increase the sensitivity to estrogen. Another link to cancer is that milk has high levels of two natural female sex hormones: estrone sulfate and progesterone. Sixty to eighty percent of consumed estrogens comes from dairy. It has been found that butter, eggs, milk, and cheese have direct links to breast, prostate, and ovarian cancers, which are all estrogen-based cancers.

Many studies have similar findings. Even though dairy is a good source of protein and calcium, it is very easy to find plant-based foods that deliver these nutrients and none of the harmful effects—and at a lower cost to the consumer and the planet.

Red Meat
Please remember, I grew up on a farm where we raised cattle and ate red meat and dairy every day, and my dad still does. This is not about being politically correct or protecting animal rights. This is about doing everything possible to beat cancer.

Harvard Medical School published a report in the *Harvard Health Publications* about two large studies done in 2005. One study followed 478 men and women who were cancer free. They found that the people who ate about 5 ounces of red meat daily had a 33 percent higher rate of colon cancer than those who didn't eat red meat or who ate less.

In another long-term study dealing with the effects of red meat consumption, 148,610 people between the ages of 50 and 74 years were followed. The study found that "a high consumption of red meats was linked with substantial increase in the risk of cancer in the lower colon and rectum."

According to the report, "a meta-analysis of 29 studies of meat consumption and colon cancer concluded that a high consumption of red meat increases risk by 28%."

In 2014, the UC San Diego School of Medicine published a study in the *Proceedings of the National Academy of Sciences* that found "feeding Neu5Gc, a sugar found only in red meat, but not in humans, increased spontaneous cancer in mice." They also found that this sugar leads to chronic inflammation in humans, with inflammation being a known cause of cancer.

The report detailed another large English study that "showed that large amounts of red meat can produce genetic damage to colon cells in just a few weeks."

And in a new study released in October 2015, the World Health Organization concludes that red meat **causes cancer**.

In all studies, "large amounts of red meat" meant anything more than 5 ounces per day. That's about the amount of beef in a standard burger.

Hydrogenated Oils and Partially Hydrogenated Oils

So, what is hydrogenated oil? Hydrogenated oil (HO) is an oil that has been processed by heating to between 500 degrees and 1,000 degrees at high atmospheric pressure. Then, a catalyst, such as nickel, platinum, or aluminum, is added that changes the molecular structure of the oil, making it denser and enabling the molecules to stay liquid at room temperature. Interestingly, the newly changed molecules have nearly the same molecular structure as the molecules in plastic!

These oils are thick, and when consumed they thicken our blood, making it harder for the heart to pump blood throughout the body. But worse than that is the damage HOs cause to the walls of the vascular system. First, they add to the buildup of plaque on the arterial walls. Also, the metal catalyst in HOs scars the walls of arteries and veins. This scarring reduces the inside diameter of the vessels and forces the heart to work harder to maintain blood flow, and less blood gets to the cells.

Studies have shown that HOs are directly related to an increased risk of Alzheimer's disease and Parkinson's disease, in part because the brain isn't getting enough blood and because of the aluminum used as a catalyst. Many studies find a link between the introduction of aluminum into the body and both diseases.

For cancer patients, the reduced blood flow brought on by the ingestion of hydrogenated oils means the body's cells are being starved of the nutrients and oxygen they need to fight off cancer and to function normally.

A study published in the *International Journal of Cancer* found that people who consumed partially hydrogenated oils (PHOs), from any source, had "increased systemic inflammation, insulin resistance and adiposity (retained fat in the body)."

A large Norwegian study on PHO done in three stages found that over the course of the study 12,004 people developed either pancreatic cancer, multiple myeloma, colon and rectal cancer, cancer of the mouth and pharynx, stomach cancer, and breast cancer.

Refined Grains

This is another hard choice to have to make because most of us like the convenience of foods made with refined grains. White bread, white rice, breakfast cereals, pasta, and pancake mix are just a few of the more popular foods made with refined grains.

Why are they on the never-eat list? Because they act exactly like sugar in the bloodstream. Refined grains are digested quickly and turn into simple sugar that is quickly absorbed into the bloodstream, causing steep spikes in blood sugar levels. Eating refined grains is the same as eating refined sugars and has the same effects on the body. Cancer patients should not eat refined grains because the excess blood sugar feeds tumor growth. For healthy people, the long-term effects are the same: elevated levels of triglycerides and cellular inflammation, which, as we know, leads to increased rates of heart disease, diabetes, and cancer. Refined grains also are a big factor in the rising obesity rates in the United States and other developed countries.

Processed Meats

This group was hard for me to give up. Like many, I love bacon, smoked hams, pepperoni, salami, and hotdogs, and, well, you get the picture. That said, we had to stop eating them because the research is overwhelming on the health risks associated with them.

The main culprits in processed meats are the multitude of preservatives used in their making. Plus, processed meats are loaded with sodium nitrites and sodium nitrates, both of which have been proven to cause cancer, especially colon and rectal cancer.

They are high in saturated fat and sodium and are very calorie dense. For example, just 1 ounce of pepperoni has 130 calories, 12 grams of total fat (which accounts for 110 calories), 4.5 grams of saturated fat, 25 milligrams of cholesterol, and 570 grams of sodium (which is about 25 percent of the recommended daily intake).

☝

We would be better off not eating many foods. But they are too numerous to list. One thing I advise anyone interested in adopting a healthier diet is to do a little research and learn about what you are putting into your body. Look up the effects all the preservatives and other added ingredients used in processed foods have on your long-term health. And remember, you must take into consideration the totality of the foods you eat because eating a little yellow dye number 5 or MSG or butylated hydroxytoluene (BHT) or brominated vegetable oil or artificial sweetener once in a while won't harm you, but the cumulative effects could be devastating. Think of it like this: one grain of sand hitting your car at 60 miles an hour leaves a microscopic mark, but when you drive through a sandstorm at 60 miles an hour, your windshield is pitted so badly you can't see out and the paint job on the windward side is completely sandblasted off.

For cancer patients and cancer survivors, the stakes are much higher. Their lives are on the line, and cancer is a relentless killer, so why would they give it any advantage by eating foods known to cause cancer or fuel its growth?

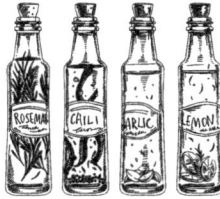

Stock Up

TO MAKE eating a plant-based diet easier, here is a list of essential foods, spices, herbs, and other items you should keep on hand. Try to buy non-GMO and organic items whenever possible.

The Spice Rack

Spices are potent cancer fighters and, as such, should be used in sufficient amounts whenever possible. This list has both pure spices along with dried herbs that function as spices. They are listed in alphabetical order rather than by cancer-fighting potency.

Allspice
Anise seed and star anise
Basil
Black pepper
Caraway
Cardamom
Cayenne pepper
Chili powder (mild, hot)
Chinese five-spice powder
Cinnamon
Clove
Coriander
Cumin
Curry
Dill

Fennel seed
Garlic powder
Ginger powder
Nutmeg (powder, bean)
Onion powder
Oregano
Paprika (Hungarian, smoked, regular)
Red pepper flakes
Rosemary
Sea salt and regular table salt with iodine
Thyme
Turmeric

Fresh Herbs
Fresh herbs are easy to grow both inside and outside the house. Having an herb garden gives you ready access to superior cancer fighters, and they add a distinctive flavor you don't get from using dried herbs. Growing your own also reduces the cost of cooking dramatically, because if you buy them at the supermarket, you can find yourself paying way too much.

Basil
Cilantro
Mint
Oregano
Parsley
Rosemary
Sage
Thyme

In the Pantry
These items include anything that can be stored at room temperature. Most are readily available at grocery stores. All these have very little or no added sugars.

Breakfast items:
Arrowhead Mills Instant Quinoa & Oat Hot Cereal
Cheerios
Hodgson Mill Buckwheat Pancake Mix
Hodgson Mill Multi Grain with Quinoa & Flax Hot Cereal
Kashi 7 Whole Grain Puffs
Oats (rolled or steel-cut; we use Bob's Red Mill)
Plant protein powder (MRM Veggie Protein powder, PlantFusion Complete Plant Protein powder, Sprouts Vegan Protein Powder, Vega One Nutritional Shake)
Shredded Wheat Biscuits
Wheat Montana Farms and Bakery Whole Grain Pancake Mix (100% whole grain, non-GMO)
Zoom cereal

Whole grains:
Barley
Brown rice
Bulgur
Popcorn
Quinoa (tricolor, red)

Legumes:
Beans (black, red, white, pinto)
Garbanzo beans, dried (chickpeas)
Lentils (green, red)

Pastas:
Ancient Harvest Lentil & Quinoa Supergrain Pasta
Ancient Harvest Supergrain Pasta
Barilla ProteinPLUS (in a limited amount as these contain some refined wheat flour)
Brown rice pasta
Soba buckwheat noodles
Whole wheat pasta

A Recipe for Hope

Canned goods:
Beans (black, red, white, vegan refried, garbanzo)
Tomatoes (fire-roasted, diced, whole)
Tomato and pasta sauces (tomato products in glass jars are better)

Flours:
Brown rice
Oat flour
Whole wheat

Sweeteners:
Organic coconut crystals (use sparingly)
Raw natural light organic 100% agave (use sparingly)
Stevia leaf or Truvia
Xylitol (powdered or Nature's Hollow Honey Substitute)

Staples:
Bananas
Dried dates and raisins
Dried mushrooms
Garlic cloves
Onions (yellow, sweet, red)
Tea (green, red, black, some herbal)
Tubers (red yams, sweet potatoes, red, and purple russets)
Vegetable broth (organic)

Nuts:
Almonds (raw, roasted)
Brazil nuts
Cashews (raw, roasted)
Peanuts (dry-roasted)
Walnuts (raw)

Things used to cook with:
Algae oil (new and exciting cooking oil)

Almond extract
Baking powder
Baking soda
Bragg Liquid Amino Acids (soy sauce substitute)
Bragg Nutritional Yeast
Bragg Organic Apple Cider Vinegar
Coconut oil
Cornstarch
Extra virgin olive oil
Vanilla extract
Vinegar (red wine, rice wine, balsamic)

In the refrigerator:
Avocados
Basil pesto spread
Bell peppers (red and green)
Capers
Carrots
Celery
Coconut milk creamer
Fresh fruits (in season is best)
Fresh ginger root
Fresh turmeric root (if you can find it)
Greens (Swiss chard, kale, mustard, spinach)
Lemons
Lettuces (red leaf, romaine, arugula, watercress)
Limes
Milk substitutes (unsweetened almond, rice, soy)
Mushrooms (brown, white, portobello, shiitake)
Mustard (Dijon, brown, yellow, whole grain)
Natural almond butter
Natural peanut butter (never use regular peanut butter as it has sugar and hydrogenated oil in them)
Radishes
Red curry paste

Sriracha sauce
Sugar-free jam (Nature's Hollow, Walden Farms, Polaner, and Smucker's all have these; however, beware of jams and jellies sweetened with fruit juice because they act like sugar in the body)
Tabasco sauce (red, green)
Tahini sauce
Tofutti milk-free sour cream (if you must, but limit your use of them)
Trader Joe's Sprouted Flourless Whole Wheat Berry Bread
Vegan butter and mayo substitutes
Yellow miso

In the freezer:
Baby peas
Blueberries
Corn
Dark cherries
Raspberries
Shredded hash brown potatoes
Spinach
Strawberries

It is a good idea to keep a few handy store-bought items that you can use in a pinch, such as Amy's Bowl Brown Rice, Black-Eyed Peas and Veggies and Amy's Light and Lean Quinoa and Black Bean with Butternut Squash and Chard. The key is to read the ingredient list carefully. Be on the lookout for what kind of oil is in a product, whether there are any added sugars, and remember, if there is an ingredient you can't pronounce or don't recognize, then it's best not to buy the item.

For those who choose to eat a little fish, look for wild-caught Alaskan salmon or cod. There are a few good frozen salmon patties that can be used as well. If you're lucky enough to live near a Trader Joe's, their Premium Salmon Burgers and Mahi Mahi Burgers are good; they also carry individual-sized frozen fresh salmon packages. It's a good idea to keep a package of tasty veggie burgers on hand too, such as Hilary's Eat Well Burgers, Organic Sunshine Harvest Burgers, or the original Boca Vegan Burgers. These brands are pretty good and aren't loaded with salt and other do-not-eat ingredients. I am including these items because there will be occasions when time is short or you just don't feel like cooking from scratch, and it's better to have a few things on hand that fit into a cancer-fighting diet than to give in to the old ways of eating. You have to think of eating like you do smoking; you can't have a cigarette just this once because that can quickly lead to a pack a day.

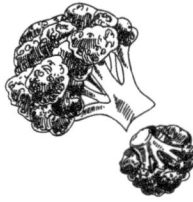

Sample Menu

WHEN CANCER patients start chemotherapy treatments for the first time, they are inundated with information about their cancer that it can be difficult to process it all. There are so many unknowns that come with cancer, such as treatment options and the effects each will have on you. New patients are hit with a flood of overwhelming emotions, especially when their cancer is advanced. Plus, there is all the outside advice cancer patients get from family and friends. Some of it may be useful, but more often than not this information is confusing or even detrimental. What's worse, many times, beyond the immediate medical aspects, patients receive little useful guidance from their medical team on how to go about their daily lives. Often missing is advice on what to eat and how important diet is to a patient's ability to live with and fight the cancer.

I can tell you it took us a long time to get our feet under us after Susan's diagnosis. One of the first obstacles we faced came the day after Susan's first chemo treatment. After beginning chemo treatments it is common for people to lose their appetite, and, sure enough, Susan started getting sick and nothing tasted good to her. One of the only diet-related suggestions we got was in our pre-chemotherapy consultations. The nurse told us that Susan couldn't eat any raw or uncooked foods because of the risk of food-born illness and infection. The risk was so high that even the slightest amount of bacteria could be deadly. To make a long story short, we were simply at a loss on what to do. We had no idea that there was a way to eat that would help in Susan's battle with cancer or even that eating certain foods would actually help promote tumor growth and weaken her immune system.

With that in mind I thought it would be a good idea to provide a sample weeklong menu for people on chemotherapy. Of course, every cancer patient would be well advised to consult with a registered dietitian with training in understanding cancer treatments and diets. Remember that every type of cancer is different, and so is every cancer patient, so that means what is right for one person may not be right for another.

This sample menu is basic, simple, and has easy-to-prepare food. It is meant as a starting point. Once we made the decision to fight Susan's cancer with food, we kept it simple and easy. We weren't trying to replicate our old diet in any way. In other words, I didn't try to make dishes that tasted like beef or chicken. Instead, I designed meals that would provide her with the right balance of nutrients and enough calories so she didn't lose too much weight, and would keep her energy levels high enough.

Monday

A glass of plant protein in 12 ounces of water or almond milk one hour before eating any carbohydrates.

Breakfast:
- Bob's Organic Oatmeal with blueberries, dark cherries, raisins, cinnamon, nutmeg and minced ginger (add the berries, raisins, and ginger during the cooking process; we use frozen berries because they are accessible year round), rice or almond milk. If you have to sweeten the cereal use Stevia or Truvia.
- A piece of sprouted wheat toast.
- An orange, thoroughly washed before peeling. Green tea.

Snack:
- Small handful of raw almonds (about 6 nuts), 1 banana.

Lunch:
- Bowl of homemade vegetable soup (heavy on the vegetables).
- A peanut butter sandwich with sugar-free jelly on whole grain bread.

- A bowl of mango or papaya with minced ginger, lime, and chili powder. Thoroughly wash the mango before peeling.
- 16 ounces of water.

Snack:

- 4 walnut halves and a small handful of sunflower seeds, unsalted.
- 16 ounces of water.

Dinner:

- Spaghetti (see food list for type and brand) with a vegan marinara sauce with lots of mushrooms and garlic (no parmesan).
- 1 large serving of steamed spinach with minced ginger and lemon (eat as much as you want and make extra for leftovers).
- 1 piece of toasted whole grain crusty bread (use Earth Balance butter substitute if you need to butter your bread).
- 16 ounces of water.

After dinner snack:

- 1 piece of citrus fruit, washed.
- A cup of Sleepytime tea before bed.

Tuesday

Breakfast:

- Chocolate protein smoothie made with 1 scoop plant protein powder, ½ cup spinach (use leftover spinach from Monday's dinner), 1 tablespoon of rolled oats, 2 teaspoons fresh minced ginger, ½ banana, 1 teaspoon ground flaxseed, 1 teaspoon unsweetened cocoa powder, 2 tablespoons frozen blueberries, steamed for 3 minutes, 8 or more ounces almond milk. Blend all the ingredients at high speed until it is well mixed.

Snack:

- Handful of roasted peanuts, unsalted.
- 16 ounces of water.

Lunch:

- Leftover spaghetti.
- Large serving of Rainbow Swiss Chard and Ginger.

→   16 ounces of water.

Snack:

→   6 almond pieces and an orange.

Dinner:

→   Cuban Black Beans and Brown Rice.

→   ½ ripe avocado.

→   Chili–lime corn (put the corn kernels in a pan over medium heat, add chili powder and lime juice).

→   Warm Red Cabbage and Green Apple Slaw.

→   16 ounces of water.

Snack:

→   ½ grapefruit.

→   A cup of Sleepytime tea before bed.

Wednesday

Protein shake one hour before breakfast.

Breakfast:

→   Bowl of shredded wheat, topped with banana and chopped walnuts.

→   Flourless sprouted wheat toast with peanut butter, green tea.

Snack:

→   Handful of pistachios.

Lunch:

→   Black Bean Veggie Tacos with brown rice, English cucumber (washed and peeled) with avocado slices and salsa.

→   Large serving of wilted spinach with lemon juice and minced ginger.

→   1 cup of green tea and 8 ounces of water.

Snack:

→   Orange.

Dinner:

→   Lemony Minty Lentils.

→   Crusty multi-grain bread.

Snack:

→   Air-popped popcorn (I put ¼ cup of popcorn in a brown paper

lunch bag, fold the top over, staple twice, then microwave on the popcorn setting).
→ A cup of Sleepytime tea before bed.

Thursday

Plant protein shake one hour before breakfast.

Breakfast:
✦ Bob's 10 Grain Cereal with minced ginger, banana slices, blueberries, ¼ teaspoon turmeric, and cinnamon.
→ ½ grapefruit.
→ Green tea.

Snack:
→ 4 walnut halves and 1 citrus fruit.

Lunch:
→ Bowl of leftover Lemony Minty Lentils, crusty bread, and 16 ounces of water.

Snack:
→ ½ peanut butter sandwich on sprouted wheat bread.

Dinner:
→ Jeff's Veggie Pizza and 16 ounces of water.

Snack:
→ Small serving of any leftovers or an orange if you don't have leftovers.
→ A cup of Sleepytime tea before bed.

Friday

Protein shake one hour before breakfast.

Breakfast:
→ Peanut butter and banana sandwich.
→ Green tea.

Snack:
→ Almonds.

Lunch:
→ Walnut and wilted spinach salad (simply wilt a big bunch of washed, fresh spinach in a sauté pan, add juice of 1 lemon

and some minced ginger and cook until spinach is thoroughly heated. Top with chopped walnuts).

Snack:

➜ ½ fresh melon (anything in season) thoroughly washed before cutting.

Dinner:

➜ This might sound strange, but make Friday night your date night. Go out to dinner somewhere where you can get a vegan meal. Check local eateries to see which ones have things on their menu you can eat, call ahead and see if the chef will accommodate special orders like no sugars, low salt content, or if they can even make a dish specially for you. You will be surprised how many of them will and they take it as a personal challenge to come up with something good. Having a date night is really important for your personal morale and you will need a break. Chemo treatments suck and they can get you down, so get out and try to enjoy yourself a little.

➜ A cup of Sleepytime tea before bed.

Saturday

Plant protein shake one hour before breakfast.

Breakfast:

➜ Breakfast Veggie Skillet with sprouted wheat toast.

➜ 1 orange.

Snack:

➜ Handful of nuts.

Lunch:

➜ Roasted Butternut Squash Soup with crusty multi-grain bread.

➜ 16 ounces of water.

Snack:

➜ Spicy Roasted Red Yam Rounds.

Dinner:

➜ Chickpeas with Fire-Roasted Tomato Sauce over brown rice (make extra and save some for later).

Snack:
- ➜ Popcorn with turmeric (heat a large saucepan and add 1 teaspoon of coconut oil, 1 teaspoon of turmeric, then ¼ cup popcorn and pop. Make sure to shake the pan a few times so as not to burn the corn kernels).
- ➜ A cup of Sleepytime tea before bed.

Sunday

Plant protein shake one hour before breakfast.

Breakfast:
- ➜ Oatmeal Pancakes with Blueberry Compote.
- ➜ ½ grapefruit.
- ➜ Green tea.

Snack:
- ➜ Handful of leftover roasted chickpeas.

Lunch:
- ➜ Large serving of sautéed rainbow Swiss chard topped with sunflower seeds.
- ➜ 16 ounces of water.

Snack:
- ➜ Diced mango with chili powder and lime (wash and peel a mango, cut the flesh from the seed and cube. In a bowl, add the mango, squeeze ½ a small lime, ⅛ teaspoon chili powder and ½ teaspoon fresh, finely minced ginger).
- ➜ 16 ounces of water.

Dinner:
- ➜ Mexican Black Bean Lasagna with Avocado and Cilantro.
- ➜ Large serving of sautéed julienned red and green bell peppers and red onion.
- ➜ 16 ounces of water.

Snack:
- ➜ A piece of a dark chocolate bar (85% cacao and sugar-free if you can find it. We have a small piece every evening as a treat).
- ➜ A cup of Sleepytime tea before bed.

One thing you may have noticed is I made sure to include water intake for each day, and that's because when someone is getting chemotherapy treatments they should drink between 64 and 82 ounces of water every day (this translates to 8 to 10 cups). I included the water as a reminder and in case the doctors don't mention it. Carry a water bottle with you all day. And eat lots of dark leafy greens (cooked, of course) and brightly colored vegetables, and avoid any sugar, white rice, or white bread. Also, I have purposely left out all the spices and the amounts here because chemo will affect your sense of taste. That said, cancer patients on chemo should try to add as much ginger, turmeric, fresh mint leaves, peppermint, cinnamon, and chamomile to their meals, as these all help with alleviating nausea. The ginger, peppermint, mint leaves, and chamomile are great when added to tea.

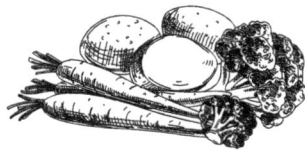

PART III

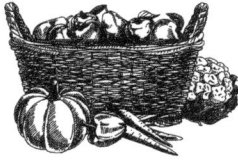

Recipes

REMEMBER THAT I'm trying to use food as medicine, so I make dishes that have known cancer-fighting ingredients. When I was developing these dishes, the goal was to load up each dish with as many and as much of the best cancer fighters as I could. Taste was secondary, but still quite important because food that doesn't taste good makes it hard to stick to the plan. Fortunately, some of the best cancer-fighting ingredients are the ingredients that make most dishes taste great, such as herbs, spices, garlic, and onions. Nuts and berries are way up there on the best-of list, too.

It's important to say that I try to keep my cooking as simple as possible. I don't have hundreds of recipes, and the ones I have are easy to cook. The key is to eat as many cancer-fighting foods as possible, not to be a gourmet chef. I like to have fun cooking and try to make it a family thing as often as I can.

When I cook, I add as much ginger root, turmeric root, turmeric powder, oregano, chili powder, cayenne pepper, garlic, and onion as I can. I don't mind experimenting with spices and herbs until I hit on recipes that we really like. Sometimes they work and sometimes they don't.

When you are cooking, start off with less and keep adding the spice or herb, tasting as you go. It's easy to tell when to stop. Write down what you have added and how much. Sometimes you hit on a perfect blend and your dish turns out really well. But, if you don't write down everything, it can be hard to replicate the dish the next time. I'm certainly guilty of this. I've failed to record recipes for a few dishes that turned out so darn good, and now I can't figure out how I made them.

Whenever possible, use organic greens and vegetables. The toxins and pesticides used in commercial farming are known to cause cancer.

These days, I don't grow many flowers; instead, I grow food. Herbs grow well in pots and can be grown year-round indoors, so try growing your own. That way, you always have them on hand for spur-of-the-moment cooking.

Outside I have an enclosed wooden planter that I grow mint in (it will take over if you don't enclose the plants). Pots full of perennial herbs, such as oregano, thyme, and sage, line my yard. Plus I have a big rosemary bush and it never needs replanting. Every empty space gets replanted with edibles that are in season, such as tomatoes, basil, cilantro, parsley, chard, or leaf lettuce.

In a small section of my backyard I grow Swiss chard and kale year round. By picking only the bigger leaves off the chard plants they keep producing new ones so I rarely have to replant. Kale will also keep growing, if you pick only the bottom leaves. I don't use pesticides, so once in a while I have to cut out bug-damaged sections of the leaves. It's not much trouble at all, especially considering the fresh taste and easy access. I also grow bell pepper plants and jalapeño peppers.

Down here in Southern California we grow citrus, which is nice because we have lemons and limes nearly year-round, and I have several semi-dwarf fruit trees for that purpose. Wherever you live, grow fruit trees that will do well in your climate. Many dwarf varieties can be grown in bigger pots, too.

I also have a network of friends and neighbors, and we all share the things we grow with each other. I trade citrus for avocados and plums. One of my neighbors has a small strip of land about three feet wide and thirty feet long that she doesn't use, so I made a deal with her. Now I grow vegetables and greens in that space and we share the crops. To save space, I grow cucumbers in a big hanging pot.

My point is there are a lot of things you can do to cut the cost of your food bill and to grow safe and fresh foods.

Beyond what I can grow, I make sure we always have spinach, blueberries, raspberries, tart cherries, and strawberries in the freezer. I make lots of smoothies for breakfast with a chocolate-flavored plant protein powder (we use PlantFusion or VegaOne), a little of each berry, banana, fresh ginger, ground flaxseed, chia seeds, and spinach. Susan has Bob's Red Mill Organic Rolled Oats for breakfast most mornings, and she tops it with a little banana, blueberry, cherries, cinnamon, clove, and nutmeg. I use the frozen spinach in any dish I think it will work in. Some other essential items to have on hand are quinoa, beans of all colors, uncooked garbanzo beans (chickpeas), brown rice, whole wheat noodles, brown rice noodles, buckwheat noodles, ground flaxseed, chia seeds, almonds, walnuts, jars of tomato sauce, and tomato paste.

Keep in mind that, when a cancer patient is getting chemotherapy treatments, everything must be thoroughly washed and cooked. No raw foods are allowed because of the threat of infections and *Salmonella*. Furthermore, hot spices can irritate the mouth and throat, so be careful.

Finally, remember that you have to stick to your routine. Fighting cancer is a full-time job and must be treated as such. Finding recipes you love will help you maintain that routine.

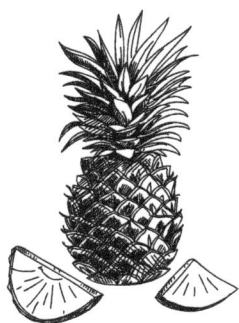

Breakfast

Oatmeal Pancakes with Blueberry Compote

Ingredients for pancake batter

¾ cup sugar-free almond milk

2 teaspoons Bragg Unfiltered Organic Apple Cider Vinegar

2 teaspoons organic coconut oil

2 tablespoons unsweetened applesauce

Pinch of nutmeg

1 teaspoon cinnamon

½ cup Bob's Red Mill Organic Rolled Oats (quick-cooking)

½ cup whole wheat flour

1 teaspoon baking powder

1 teaspoon baking soda

¼ teaspoon salt

Ingredients for blueberry compote

¾ cup blueberries, fresh or frozen

½ cup water

1 teaspoon lemon juice

1 teaspoon fresh ginger root, grated

¼ teaspoon vanilla extract

1 tablespoon cornstarch

Preparation

For the pancake batter, combine almond milk, vinegar, coconut oil, applesauce, nutmeg, and cinnamon in a medium-sized mixing bowl. Add the oats and soak for 5 minutes.

In a separate mixing bowl, sift whole wheat flour, baking powder, and baking soda, then add salt. Slowly, add the dry mixture to the wet mixture, and stir until well incorporated. Set aside.

For the blueberry compote, add all the ingredients except the cornstarch into a small saucepan over medium-low heat for 5 minutes, stirring occasionally. Put a tablespoon of cornstarch in a small bowl and add a little water, stirring

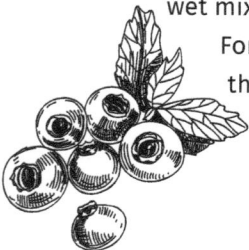

until cornstarch is smooth. Add the cornstarch mixture to the blueberries, mixing slowly until the sauce thickens. Remember, the sauce must come to a slow boil before it thickens. If it becomes too thick, add water until you get the sauce to the desired consistency. It should pour easily.

To make the pancakes, preheat a large, non-stick skillet over medium heat. Ladle the pancake batter into the pan to make 4-inch cakes. Cook for 2 to 3 minutes, until bubbles form on the top. Lift the sides of the cakes to check for an even-brown color, then flip. Cook for an additional 1 to 2 minutes. Serve with the blueberry compote drizzled over the pancakes.

Breakfast Veggie Skillet

Ingredients

3 medium-sized red or purple potatoes, cubed
1 tablespoon extra-virgin olive oil or coconut oil
½ red onion, diced
1 teaspoon fresh rosemary, chopped finely
1 teaspoon dried oregano
1 small broccoli floret, segmented
1 cup chopped spinach, fresh or frozen (thawed)
1 cup portobello mushrooms, sliced
½ red bell pepper, diced
½ green bell pepper, diced
¼ teaspoon sea salt
⅛ teaspoon ground black pepper
⅛ teaspoon garlic powder
⅛ cup fresh parsley or cilantro, chopped
Pinch of cayenne pepper (careful with this, it's easy to go overboard)

Preparation

Place the potatoes in a medium saucepan partially filled with water and bring to boil, cooking until fork-tender, 12 to 15 minutes. Be sure not to overcook them. Drain the water and set aside. Heat the olive oil in a large cast-iron skillet over medium heat, then add the potatoes and cook until they start to brown. Add onion, rosemary, and dried oregano and toss. Add broccoli and cook for about 2 minutes, then add the spinach and mushrooms. Sauté for 3 to 4 minutes, turning the ingredients over once or twice. Add the red and green bell peppers, then sprinkle on the sea salt, ground black pepper, garlic powder, and cayenne pepper. Turn off the heat, add the chopped herbs, and mix everything together. Serve with your favorite salsa as a topping.

Breakfast Veggie Sandwich with Cashew Hollandaise Sauce

Ingredients
4 whole wheat English muffins
4 thick tomato slices
1 avocado, peeled and sliced
¼ cup fresh basil, chopped roughly

Hollandaise Sauce
1 cup raw cashews, soaked
2 teaspoons Dijon mustard
1 lemon, zested and juiced
1 teaspoon garlic powder
½ teaspoon turmeric powder
Paprika and cayenne pepper to taste
1 teaspoon nutritional yeast
½ cup warm water

Preparation
To make the hollandaise sauce, bring 1½ cups of water to boil. Add cashews and simmer for 10 minutes, then drain. Put the softened

cashews, mustard, lemon zest and juice, garlic powder, turmeric, paprika, cayenne pepper, nutritional yeast, and ½ cup warm water in a blender and puree until smooth, about 1 minute. Add more water to get the right consistency. The sauce will keep for three days if refrigerated in an airtight container.

To prepare the sandwiches, split and toast the wheat muffins. Put a tomato slice and some avocado slices on the muffins, pour a little hollandaise sauce over the sandwich, and top with fresh chopped basil

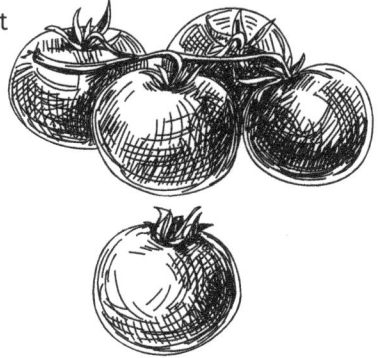

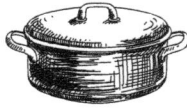

Soups

Roasted Butternut Squash Soup

Ingredients

1 butternut squash

1 Granny Smith apple

1 medium yellow onion

1 tablespoon extra-virgin olive oil

1 teaspoon sea salt

⅛ teaspoon black pepper

5 cups vegetable broth

½ teaspoon turmeric

½ teaspoon cinnamon

Pinch of cayenne pepper (careful, too much will
make the soup too spicy)

¼ teaspoon fresh thyme, chopped finely

½ teaspoon fresh rosemary, chopped finely

⅛ teaspoon grated nutmeg

2 tablespoons coconut sugar or 3 dates, soaked and pureed

Preparation

Preheat oven to 375°F. Peel and cube the squash. Quarter and take out the seed part of the apple. Quarter the onion and run a toothpick through each section to hold it together.

Put the squash cubes, apple, and onion in a large mixing bowl, drizzle with olive oil and toss. Spread the cubes out on two trays lined with foil or parchment paper, salt and pepper to taste, and roast them at 375°F for 30 to 35 minutes, tossing them a couple times so they start to brown on all sides.

Put the roasted veggies in a food processor, or a food mill if you have one, and process them until they become a thick puree. Next, transfer a couple cups of the puree to a blender, taking care not to overfill it, and add veggie broth a little at a time as you blend until achieving a

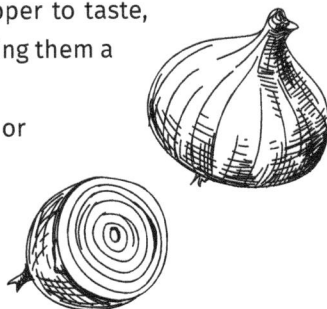

nice smooth mixture. Pour the mixture into a large pot, repeating the blending process until all the puree has been used. Add the rest of the vegetable broth to the pot. Add the herbs and spices.

As the soup is warming, add the pureed dates until you get the desired sweetness. Simmer for 15 minutes.

Mainly White Bean and Kale Soup

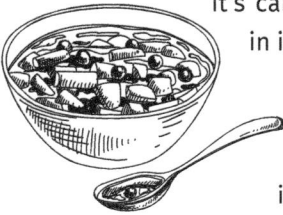

It's called "mainly" because white beans are plentiful in it, but there are other types of beans as well. This was something I came up with because I wanted to see how many cancer-fighting ingredients I could put in one dish. Turns out quite a few, and it tastes really good.

Ingredients
1 cup dry white beans
½ cup Bob's Red Mill 13-Bean Mix
4 cups vegetable broth
½ cup onion, chopped
1 clove garlic, minced
8-oz can diced or fire-roasted tomatoes
2 cups kale, chopped
1 cup red cabbage, shredded and chopped
½ cup portobello mushrooms, chopped
1 carrot, chopped
Zest and juice of 1 lemon and lemon
wedges to serve

Spices
1 teaspoon dried oregano
¼ teaspoon turmeric
½ teaspoon chili powder
½ teaspoon cumin

¼ teaspoon smoked paprika
¼ teaspoon dried mustard
Pinch of cayenne pepper
2 teaspoons sea salt or to taste (start with 1 teaspoon
and season again later)
⅛ teaspoon black pepper

Preparation

Put beans in a large pot the night before and cover with water, making sure the water is 2 inches higher than the level of the beans. Soak overnight. Alternatively, if you have the time day of, add water to cover the bean mix to a level about 2 inches above the beans, then bring it to a boil. Turn the heat down to simmer for 1 hour or so until the beans are almost cooked. Drain the water and set the beans aside.

Add a little broth to the pot and sauté the onions on low heat for 2 minutes. Mix all the spices in a small bowl. Add the spice mixture to the pot and sauté another 2 minutes. Add the minced garlic. Return the bean mix to the pot. Pour in the remaining vegetable broth, making sure there are a couple inches of broth covering the bean mix. Add the diced tomatoes and cook for 30 minutes. Add the kale, red cabbage, mushrooms, and carrots and simmer for 30 minutes or until the beans are tender. Check to see whether you need more salt as the beans cook. (Test them every 15 minutes to be sure they are done, but not overcooked.)

When the beans are tender and you are satisfied with the seasoning, turn off the heat and add the juice and zest of 1 lemon, cover, and let stand for 10 to 15 minutes. Serve with a nice crusty whole wheat bread and a squeeze of lemon juice over each serving.

Lemony Minty Lentils

Ingredients

2 teaspoons extra-virgin olive oil

1 red onion, diced

2 cloves garlic, minced

4 cups vegetable broth

¾ cup green lentils

¼ cup red lentils

4 red or purple potatoes, diced

1 carrot, chopped

½ cup portobello mushrooms, chopped

Zest and juice of 1 lemon and lemon wedges to serve

1 bunch flat-leaf kale or rainbow Swiss chard or one 16-oz package frozen spinach, chopped

½ cup or more fresh mint, chopped

Spices

1 teaspoon sea salt

¼ teaspoon black pepper

Pinch of cayenne pepper

½ teaspoon cumin

½ teaspoon turmeric

½ teaspoon coriander powder

½ teaspoon chili powder

¼ teaspoon smoked paprika

Preparation

In a large pot over medium heat, add olive oil and diced onion and sauté for 2 minutes. Add the garlic and spices and cook for 1 minute more. Add the broth, green lentils, red lentils, potatoes, carrots, and mushrooms. Cover and simmer for 15 to 20 minutes. The lentils and potatoes should be tender. Check broth level occasionally and add more as needed.

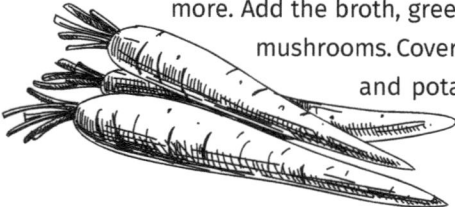

274

Zest the lemon, finely mince the zest, and add it, along with the greens, and cook for about 4 minutes. Add the juice of the lemon and the mint and stir well. Cook for 2 more minutes.

To serve, squeeze a wedge of lemon on the dish to brighten it. Serve with warm whole wheat bread.

Rosemary 13-Bean Soup

Ingredients
1 cup Bob's Red Mill 13-Bean mix
1 small yellow onion, diced
¼ cup shiitake mushrooms, diced
½ cup portobello mushrooms, diced
1 quart water
1 14-oz can fire-roasted tomatoes
1 cup vegetable broth
¼ cup green bell pepper, diced
1 carrot, diced
Zest of 1 lemon
1 cup red cabbage, shredded
Juice of 1 lemon
2 tablespoons apple cider vinegar

Spices
1 teaspoon sea salt
⅛ teaspoon black pepper
½ teaspoon cumin
½ teaspoon coriander powder
¼ teaspoon smoked paprika
1 teaspoon chili powder
1 teaspoon garlic powder
1 teaspoon dried oregano
1 teaspoon dried thyme
2 teaspoons fresh rosemary, minced finely

Preparation

In a large pot, cover beans completely with water and soak overnight, or the day of, cover beans with water and bring to a boil for 2 minutes, cover the pot, and soak for 1 hour.

Drain and rinse the soaked beans and set aside. Over medium-high heat, add diced onion and mushrooms to the pot and cook for 2 minutes. Add all the dry spices and cook for another 2 minutes. Add the beans back to the pot along with 1 quart of water, add the fire-roasted tomatoes and vegetable broth, cook for 5 minutes, then place heat on low and add the diced green bell peppers, diced carrot, fresh herbs, lemon zest, and red cabbage. Simmer for 15 to 20 minutes or until beans are tender. Make sure the water level does not drop below the top of the beans; add more water if needed. Add the lemon juice and apple cider vinegar, turn off the flame, and let the pot sit for 5 to 10 minutes.

Serve with toasted, crusty whole wheat baguette and a mixed-greens salad with avocado, cucumber, red bell pepper, and a balsamic vinaigrette dressing.

Cuban Black Beans and Brown Rice

Ingredients

1½ cups dry black beans or 2 15-oz cans black beans, rinsed

1 cup uncooked long-grain brown rice

1 bunch cilantro, chopped, reserving 1 tablespoon for serving

1 yellow onion, diced

1 green bell pepper, diced

2 garlic cloves, minced finely

1 tablespoon apple cider vinegar

Zest and juice of 1 lime

1 avocado

Spices
2 bay leaves
1½ teaspoons cumin
1 teaspoon chili powder
1 teaspoon oregano
½ teaspoon smoked paprika
¼ teaspoon cinnamon
1 teaspoon sea salt
⅛ teaspoon black pepper
Pinch of cayenne pepper

Preparation
If using dry beans, the night before put the dry beans in a large pot and cover the beans with water (well over the beans). Bring to boil, then turn off the heat, cover, and soak overnight. Cook the brown rice per instructions on the rice packaging. After the rice is cooked, add a ¼ cup finely chopped cilantro and mix.

In a large pot over medium heat, drizzle a little extra-virgin olive oil, add half of the diced onions and all of the diced green bell peppers, and sauté for 2 minutes. Add minced garlic and sauté for 1 more minute. Add the black beans and cover with water. Add all the spices. Heat to near boiling, then reduce heat to a low simmer and cook covered for 30 minutes. Check water level and make sure it stays about level with the beans.

When the beans are nice and tender, add the apple cider vinegar and the zest and juice of the lime, stir, cover, and let sit for 10 minutes.

To serve, place ½ cup of cooked brown rice in a good-sized bowl, then add 1 cup of the black beans. Top it with 1 tablespoon of diced avocado, some finely diced onion, and the remaining tablespoon of chopped cilantro.

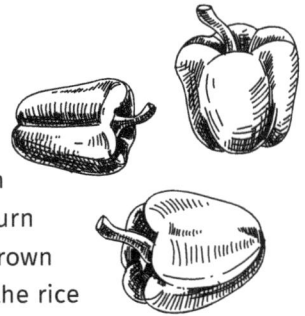

Mushroom Pho with Bok Choy

Ingredients

1 32-oz carton of organic vegetable broth
1 small yellow onion, halved and sliced
1 clove garlic, minced
⅛ cup dried mushrooms, shiitake/porcini
1 teaspoon fresh ginger root, chopped finely
2 whole star anise
⅛ teaspoon anise seed
⅛ teaspoon ground cumin
Pinch of black pepper
¼ teaspoon sea salt
¼ teaspoon celery powder
¼ teaspoon coriander powder
½ teaspoon Chinese five-spice powder
1 tablespoon Bragg Liquid Aminos
1 cup brown crimini mushrooms, sliced
¼ cup white mushrooms, sliced
Zest of 1 lime and lime slices to serve
1 12-oz package Japanese udon noodles or buckwheat noodles
2 small bunches of bok choy, washed and chopped
¼ cup cilantro, chopped
¼ cup green onion tops, chopped

Preparation

Heat a large pot over medium heat and add 1 tablespoon of the vegetable broth and the sliced onions and sauté until they start to brown slightly, 5 to 10 minutes (this gives a nice sweet flavor). Add minced garlic and cook for 1 minute more. Add the rest of the broth and the diced dried mushrooms, minced ginger, and all the spices. Cook for 5 minutes and reduce heat to simmer. Add the liquid

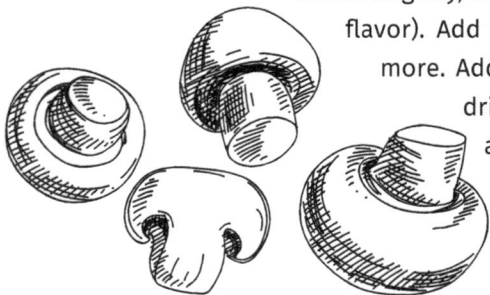

aminos. Taste and add more spices to your liking (usually Chinese five-spice powder and liquid amino will bring up a more vibrant flavor). Simmer for 10 minutes, then add the sliced mushrooms and lime zest and simmer for another 15 minutes. As the broth simmers, bring a large pot of water to boil and cook the noodles per package instructions. When done, drain and rinse. Add the bok choy to the broth and turn off the heat. I usually like to add a few small broccoli florets when I add bok choy. Don't cook this too long; just let the hot broth warm the vegetables up.

To serve, put some noodles in a large soup bowl and add the broth and veggies. Top with some chopped cilantro, green onions, and the juice of a slice of lime. If you want to kick this recipe up, squeeze in 2 to 4 drops of Sriracha sauce or add a few thin slices of fresh jalapeño pepper, or to really kick it up, add both and enjoy this dish spicy hot.

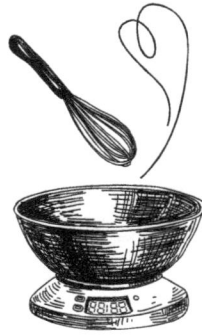

Wraps, Pizzas, and Tacos

Black Bean Veggie Tacos

(Use the recipe for the Cuban Black Beans and Brown Rice.) This is a great meal that uses up leftover black beans and rice.

Ingredients
Yellow corn tortillas
Brown rice, cooked
Black beans
English cucumber, cut into tortilla-length slices ¼ inch thick
1 lime, in wedges
Louisiana hot sauce or some green Tabasco
1 avocado, diced
¼ sweet onion, diced finely
1 tomato, diced
¼ cup cilantro, chopped
1 cup fresh spinach, chopped

Preparation
Prepare Cuban Black Beans and Brown Rice or use leftovers.

Chop all the veggies and slice the cucumber. Heat the corn tortillas over the flame of a gas burner until they start to turn color in a few spots or just heat them up so they are pliable. To build the tacos, put about a tablespoon of brown rice on the tortilla and add a tablespoon of black beans. Place a slice of cucumber on each side of the rice and beans. Squeeze a wedge of lime over the beans. Splash on a little Louisiana hot sauce or some green Tabasco (my favorite), and add the diced avocado, onion, and tomato. Top with the chopped cilantro and chopped spinach. These are so good.

Jeff's Veggie Pizza

Ingredients

1 head garlic

2 8-oz cans tomato sauce

1 teaspoon oregano

1 teaspoon garlic powder

1 teaspoon dried Italian seasoning

1 small eggplant

1 small yellow onion

2 ripe tomatoes

1 package of whole wheat pita bread or whole wheat Arabic bread rounds

1 cup fresh basil, chopped

1 tablespoon sun-dried tomatoes, chopped

1 large portobello mushroom

1 6.5-oz jar Mezzetta marinated artichoke hearts

½ cup sliced black olives

¼ cup Kalamata olives, sliced

Preparation

Roast the head of garlic by cutting it in half and drizzling a tiny bit of extra-virgin olive oil over each half. Wrap the halves in a foil pouch and bake at 350°F for 15 minutes. Take out of the oven and set aside. Turn heat up to 410°F to bake pizza.

Make the pizza sauce in a nonstick frying pan over low heat. Add the tomato sauce, oregano, garlic powder, and Italian seasoning and simmer for 15 minutes. The sauce should be semi-thick, but not paste-like.

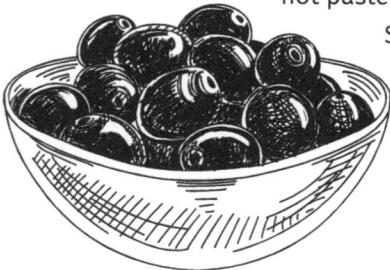

Slice the eggplant into ¼-inch rounds and grill in a cast-iron pan until they color. Slice the onion into thin rounds, then halve them. Thinly slice the tomatoes.

To build the pizza, place three pita bread

282

rounds on a pizza baking tin. Spread some sauce on top of the pitas. Spread a little chopped basil on top of the sauce and then sprinkle on the chopped sun-dried tomatoes. Put one layer of sliced tomatoes followed by one layer of grilled eggplant. Slice the portobello mushrooms from top to underside, ¼ inch thick, and layer on top of the eggplant. Layer the onions on next, making sure to use plenty of them as they will cook down. Next, cut the quartered artichoke hearts in half and spread them around. Squeeze the roasted garlic cloves from their skins and spread around on pizzas. Layer on the black and Kalamata olives. Place the pizza pan in the oven and bake for 12 minutes.

Black Bean Lentil Wrap

Ingredients for Bean and Lentil Mix
½ cup dry red lentils
1 15-oz can black beans, rinsed
1 teaspoon cumin
1 teaspoon chili powder
½ teaspoon Chinese five-spice powder
½ teaspoon turmeric
½ teaspoon sea salt
⅛ teaspoon black pepper
Pinch of cayenne pepper
1 teaspoon garlic powder
1 teaspoon onion powder
3 tablespoons lemon juice
1 tablespoon lemon zest

-

Whole wheat or multigrain wraps
¼ cup mint leaves, chopped
Bean sprouts
1 cup spinach
¼ cup jicama, diced

½ cup cucumber, diced
2 tablespoons red or sweet onion, diced finely

Dipping sauce
¼ cup yellow miso
2 tablespoons sesame ginger vinaigrette
2 tablespoons Trader Joe's Island Soyaki (it's a teriyaki sauce with pineapple juice, ginger, sesame seeds)
2 teaspoons lemon juice
4 drops of sriracha sauce
Pinch of salt and pepper

Preparation
In a small saucepan, bring 1 cup water to boil. Add red lentils, reduce heat, and cook for 10 minutes or until lentils are tender. Set aside to cool. When lentils are cooled, place them in a food processor along with the rinsed black beans and pulse to a semi-loose paste. You may need to add some veggie broth to loosen the mix. Add the cumin, chili powder, five-spice, turmeric, salt, pepper, cayenne pepper, garlic powder, onion powder, lemon juice, and zest and pulse until spices are thoroughly mixed in. Taste as you go—you may want to add a little more of one or more of the spices. You can add some Thai peanut sauce to the mixture as well, and this makes a nice variation.

To make the dipping sauce, combine miso in a small bowl with the other ingredients, tasting as you go. The sauce should be the consistency of tomato sauce.

Heat a large pan and warm the multigrain wraps so they are pliable. Place a heated wrap on a cutting board and spread 3 or 4 tablespoons of the bean-lentil mix, then add condiments (mint, bean sprouts, spinach, jicama, cucumber, onion). Cut in half, serve with dipping sauce, and enjoy.

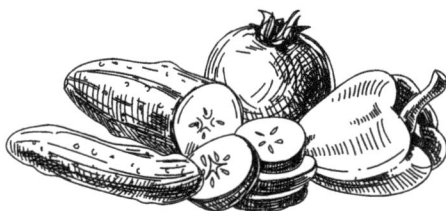

Salads

Salads are a big part of our diet because we can get so many low-fat and low-calorie ingredients in them and they are packed with cancer-fighting nutrients. The key is to add lots of red, yellow, and orange bell peppers, radishes, red onion, mushrooms, carrots, chickpeas, and black beans whenever you can. Always use organic greens and use as many varieties as you want. Try making your own salad dressing; it's not hard and you can avoid all the additives and preservatives in bottled dressing. Or, if you're pressed for time, just squeeze a little lemon and lime juice on. I also grind some black pepper on all my salads. If you're not sure where to start with a dressing, the first recipe in this section is one I make often.

Ginger Citrus Dressing

Ingredients
¼ cup extra-virgin olive oil
½ lemon
¼ lime
1 section grapefruit
2 teaspoons fresh ginger root, grated
½ teaspoon lemon zest
Pinch of sea salt
Pinch of black pepper
Pinch of cayenne pepper
Pinch of garlic powder

Preparation
Pour all the ingredients in a small mixing bowl and whisk vigorously until emulsified.

Lemony Kale Salad

Ingredients
1 bunch of organic curly-leaf kale
2 tablespoons extra-virgin olive oil
2 tablespoons fresh lemon juice
¼ teaspoon sea salt
Pinch of cayenne pepper

Preparation
Strip the leafy parts of the kale from the stems, which are tough, and chop or tear the leaves into small bite-sized pieces. Put them into a large mixing bowl. Make the dressing by putting the extra-virgin olive oil in a bowl and drizzling in the lemon juice while whisking. Add the salt and a pinch of cayenne pepper and whisk a

little more until you get a smooth emulsion. Dress the kale with the emulsion and toss a few times to coat the kale. This salad will keep for a day or two in the refrigerator.

Kale Quinoa Salad with Avocado

Ingredients
½ cup red quinoa
1 bunch curly-leaf kale
1 ripe avocado
Juice of ½ a lemon
¼ cup cilantro, chopped
¼ teaspoon garlic powder
¼ chili powder
1 teaspoon sea salt
Pinch of black pepper
1 tablespoon fresh ginger, grated
1 bunch radishes, sliced

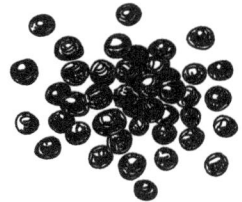

Preparation
Make the quinoa ahead of time according to the package's directions and let it cool. De-stem and tear the kale leaves into bite-sized pieces and put them in a large mixing bowl. In a smaller mixing bowl, mash the peeled and seeded avocado. Add the juice of ½ a lemon or more, depending on your preference, the cilantro and spices, salt, and pepper. Microplane or grate the fresh ginger into the avocado mixture and, with a fork, mix all the ingredients together. It should be kind of thick; if it's too loose, add a little more avocado.

Add the avocado mix to the kale and mix using your hands as if you were massaging the leaves. This will help break down the kale while thoroughly coating it with the dressing. Add the quinoa and radishes and mix everything together.

Warm Brussels Sprouts and Chickpea Salad

Ingredients
2 tablespoons extra-virgin olive oil
1 pound Brussels sprouts, trimmed and sliced thinly
¼ cup onion, sliced thinly
1 clove garlic, minced
1 15-oz can chickpeas, rinsed and drained
⅓ cup walnuts, chopped
Zest and juice of 1 lemon
1 tablespoon rice vinegar
Salt and pepper

Spices
¼ teaspoon turmeric
¼ teaspoon cardamom
¼ teaspoon coriander

Preparation
Heat 1 tablespoon of olive oil in a frying pan and add the thinly sliced Brussels sprouts and onion slices. Sauté over medium heat for 3 minutes. Add garlic and cook for 1 minute. Empty the pan into a large serving or mixing bowl.

Returning the frying pan to medium heat, add 1 tablespoon extra-virgin olive oil, add the rinsed chickpeas and chopped walnuts, and sauté until slightly toasted, about 1 minute. Stir a few times so as not to burn them. Then add the spices and lemon zest and cook 1 minute more. Add the chickpea mixture to the serving bowl, and then add the vinegar, lemon juice, and salt and pepper to taste. You can adjust the seasoning by adding more lemon juice or rice vinegar.

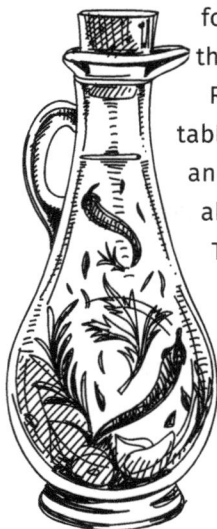

Roasted Beet and Tomato Salad

Ingredients

1 large beet
1 ripe tomato, seeded and cubed
1 cup cherry tomatoes, halved and seeded
2 tablespoons extra-virgin olive oil
Sea salt and black pepper
Juice of ½ a small lemon
¼ cup basil, chopped
¼ cup cilantro, chopped

Preparation

Heat oven to 350° F. Scrub the beet and cut into ½-inch cubes. Cut one large tomato and all the cherry tomatoes in half and seed them. Put the beet cubes and tomatoes in a large mixing bowl with 1 tablespoon of olive oil and toss. Add salt and pepper to taste. Pepper is a cancer fighter, whereas salt is not, so try to use less salt and as much pepper as you can. Line a cookie sheet with parchment paper and spread the beets on one half of the cookie sheet and tomatoes on the other half, making sure the tomatoes are skin side down. Roast for 20 minutes, turning the vegetables once. Remove the tomatoes from the sheet, turn the beets again, and roast for another 5 minutes.

While the beets and tomatoes are roasting, whisk together 1 tablespoon of olive oil and the juice of ½ a small lemon until emulsified. Put the cubed fresh tomato in a serving bowl along with the roasted cherry tomatoes. When the beets are roasted, put them in the mixing bowl to cool. When they are cooled, add them to the serving bowl with the tomatoes. Add the dressing, basil, and cilantro and toss.

Mixed Greens and Strawberry Watermelon Salad

Ingredients

About 2 oz each of baby chard, spinach,
arugula, and radicchio
½ cup cucumber, diced
½ cup red bell pepper, diced
½ ripe avocado, cubed
¼ cup ripe tomato, diced
½ cup ripe strawberries, sliced
½ cup grapefruit, cubed
¼ cup walnuts, toasted
¼ cup blueberries
1 teaspoon fresh ginger root, grated
Balsamic vinaigrette dressing
Mint leaves, chopped

Preparation

Add the greens to a large mixing bowl (you can find prewashed and organic bags of mixed greens at most grocery stores) with all the other ingredients and toss. Lightly dress with the balsamic vinaigrette dressing and top with chopped mint.

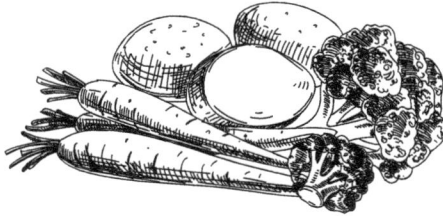

Greens and Vegetable Sides Dishes

This category should make up the largest part of your diet. These side dishes are generally easy to make, too, such as steamed broccoli, steamed asparagus, corn on the cob, wilted spinach with lemon, sautéed zucchini and yellow squash, baked acorn and butternut squash. The list is long, and it pays to eat as much of these foods as you can. Doing so helps lower your food bill, and these are among the best cancer-fighting foods.

Rainbow Swiss Chard and Ginger

Ingredients

1 bunch organic rainbow Swiss chard
¼ cup onion, thinly sliced
1 tablespoon ginger, minced
¼ cup vegetable broth
¼ teaspoon turmeric
Zest and juice of 1 lemon

Preparation

Rinse and chop the Swiss chard. Slice the onion and halve the slices. Finely mince the ginger, leaving the skin on. In a large pot over medium heat, add the broth and onion. Sauté for 2 minutes, and then add the ginger and turmeric. Add the chopped chard and cover. Zest the lemon and add both zest and juice to chard while it is cooking. Cook until the leaves are wilted, about 5 minutes.

Warm Red Peppers and Onion

Ingredients

1 red onion, halved and sliced
1 red bell pepper, julienned
Juice of ¼ lemon
Sea salt and black pepper

Preparation

Place a frying pan over medium-low heat and drizzle in 2 teaspoons extra-virgin olive oil. Add the onions and red bell peppers and sauté for no more than 2 minutes, just long enough to cook them slightly. Remove from heat and squeeze ¼ of a lemon's juice on it. Salt and pepper to taste. Serve right away. This is a great side dish for many meals; you can't have too much of this.

Warm Red Cabbage and Green Apple Slaw

Ingredients

1 tablespoon vegetable broth

½ teaspoon fresh ginger root, grated

¼ teaspoon caraway seed

¼ red onion, sliced thinly

¼ head red cabbage, sliced thinly and chopped

1 Granny Smith apple, halved and sliced

Juice of ¼ lemon

¼ cup cilantro, chopped

1 tablespoon apple cider vinegar

Sea salt and black pepper

Preparation

Heat a frying pan over medium heat. Add 1 tablespoon of vegetable broth and the ginger root, caraway seed, and onion, and cook for 1 minute. Add the cabbage and apple slices. Toss and cook for 2 minutes. Remove from the heat, add the lemon juice, apple cider vinegar, and cilantro, and toss. Add salt and pepper to taste.

Spicy Quinoa and Black Bean Salad

Ingredients

1 cup rainbow quinoa, thoroughly rinsed and cooked

2 limes

2 teaspoons ground cumin

1 teaspoon fresh ginger, minced

2 tablespoons extra-virgin olive oil

¼ teaspoon garlic powder

Pinch of cayenne pepper

Pinch of red pepper flakes

½ cup fresh, cooked, or frozen corn

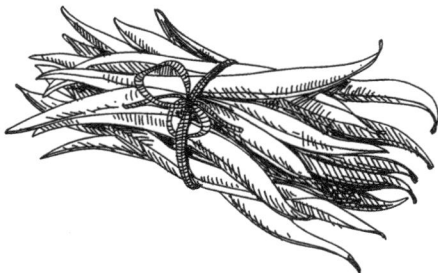

kernels
1 teaspoon chili powder
1 15-oz can black beans, drained and rinsed
1 cup cherry tomatoes, halved, or 1 cup deseeded vine-ripened tomatoes
⅛ cup green onions, finely chopped
⅓ cup cilantro, chopped
¼ teaspoon sea salt and black pepper (each)
½ teaspoon Tajín Classico Seasoning

Preparation

Cook the quinoa per package instructions. Make sure all the water is absorbed, then set aside to cool. Make the dressing in a small bowl by adding the olive oil, the juice of 1½ limes, cumin, ginger, garlic powder, cayenne pepper, and red pepper flakes and whisking thoroughly; set aside. Heat a drizzle of olive oil in a small skillet over medium heat, and add the corn kernels, cooking for 2 minutes. Then, add the chili powder and the juice of ½ a lime and toss.

In a large mixing bowl, combine the quinoa, black beans, tomatoes, chili corn, and green onions and toss. Add the dressing and toss again until well coated. Add the chopped cilantro, sea salt, black pepper, and Tajín seasoning and toss until well mixed. Taste, and if you want it a little spicier, add more cayenne pepper and taste until you get it to the spice level you want. Serve or chill and serve later.

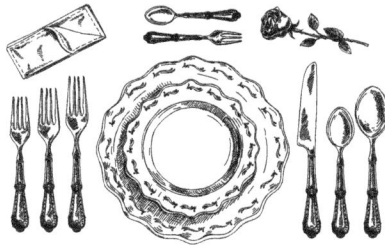

Main Dishes

Main dishes are where you can really get creative with herbs and spices. Add them to everything a little at a time, experimenting with different combinations of foods. You will be surprised at how good some of your creations are. Have fun and make it a family thing.

Jeff's Warm Red Peppers Stuffed with Cool Good Things

Ingredients

1 cup dry quinoa (makes about 2 cups cooked)
3 tablespoons extra-virgin olive oil
Juice of 1 lemon
Zest of ½ lemon
½ teaspoon garlic powder
Pinch of cayenne pepper or ½ teaspoon Miravalle Pico De Gallo seasoning (love this stuff!)
½ teaspoon sea salt
⅛ teaspoon black pepper
2 tablespoons fresh ginger, minced
2 medium tomatoes, deseeded and diced
½ cup cucumber (more if you like), diced
½ large red pepper, diced
¼ cup Mediterranean olives, diced
½ cup fresh spinach, chopped
½ cup or more mint, chopped
¼ cup parsley and a little cilantro for more flavor, chopped
2 large red peppers
⅓ cup red onion, finely diced

Preparation

Make the quinoa approximately an hour ahead of time so that it can cool down. I use red and white quinoa and don't follow the cooking instructions on the package exactly. Instead, I toast the quinoa first because it imparts a rich, nutty flavor. After it's toasted, I cook it as directed on the package.

While the quinoa is cooking, make the dressing. In a bowl, add 3 tablespoons of extra-virgin olive oil, the juice of one lemon, zest of ½ a lemon, garlic powder, cayenne pepper, sea salt, black pepper, and minced ginger. Whisk until mixture is emulsified. Pro-tip: you don't have to peel ginger; the skin has lots of flavor and you'll never know it's in your dishes.

Dice the cucumbers, ½ a red pepper, Mediterranean olives, and tomatoes. Chop the spinach, mint, and parsley and place these in a bowl and refrigerate.

After the quinoa has cooled, add the red onion and mix well and let cool. After it has cooled, fluff it and pour the dressing on. Use a fork to stir in the dressing until all the grains are coated. Let this sit for about 15 minutes so the quinoa absorbs all those wonderful flavors.

Preheat an oven to 375°F. Cut 2 red peppers from top to bottom, seed them, and remove as much of the "walls" as possible. I leave the stems on and cut them in half too because that looks pretty on the plate.

Lightly coat the pepper halves with olive oil and lightly salt and pepper them. Enclose the peppers in a foil pouch and bake for 15 to 20 minutes. The peppers should be warm and tender with a little crunch to them. Do not overcook them.

When the peppers finish cooking, mix the cucumbers, raw red peppers, Mediterranean olives, tomatoes, spinach, mint, and parsley into the quinoa. Plate the cooked pepper halves and then fill the warm halves with the cool quinoa mixture. You can top this with some crumbled vegan feta cheese to really enhance the flavor.

This is meant as a fresh and flavorful dish, so resist the urge to cook the filling with the peppers.

Chickpeas with Fire-Roasted Tomato Sauce

Ingredients
1 cup uncooked brown rice
1 15-oz can chickpeas (garbanzo beans), rinsed
1 teaspoon uncooked extra-virgin olive or coconut oil
1 small yellow onion, diced
1 cup portobello mushrooms, sliced

¼ cup shiitake mushrooms, sliced
¼ cup green bell pepper, diced
¼ cup red bell pepper, diced
1 carrot, scrubbed and sliced
1 14.5-oz jar or can fire-roasted tomatoes
½ cup vegetable broth
Zest of 1 lemon
Juice of 1 lemon
¼ cup flat-leaf parsley, chopped
1 lemon cut into wedges

Spices
½ teaspoon cumin
½ teaspoon chili powder
¼ teaspoon smoked paprika
¼ teaspoon cardamom
¼ teaspoon garlic powder
1 clove minced garlic
½ teaspoon sea salt
⅛ teaspoon black pepper
Pinch of cayenne pepper (optional)

Preparation
Preheat oven to 375°F and make the brown rice per instructions on the package.

Next, rinse and drain the chickpeas, then place them in a small mixing bowl and toss with a small amount of extra-virgin olive oil. Season the chickpeas with the following spices by shaking them on like you are salting food (these are separate from the spices listed above in the ingredients): cumin, smoked paprika, chili powder, sea salt, cardamom, and black pepper. Spread the seasoned chickpeas on a baking sheet lined with parchment paper. Roast them for 20 minutes, stirring a couple times, until they have a nice crunch.

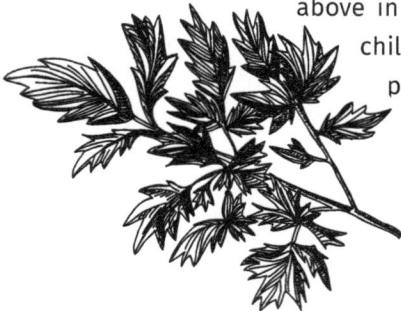

In a large frying pan over medium heat, add 1 teaspoon olive or coconut oil, sliced onion, and all the measured spices and cook for 1 minute. Add mushrooms, red and green bell peppers, and carrot and cook for 1 minute more. Then, add the fire-roasted tomatoes and the vegetable broth. Turn the heat to low, cover, and simmer for 15 minutes. At the 10-minute mark, add the roasted spicy chickpeas and lemon zest. Add extra broth as needed so the dish has enough liquid left as a sauce. Before you turn off the heat, add the lemon juice and chopped parsley. Serve over brown rice with a wedge of lemon on the side.

Toasted Coconut and Curried Rice

Ingredients
1 cup brown rice, toasted
⅓ cup coconut flakes, toasted
1 tablespoon vegan Earth Balance Butter (this is a butter substitute found at most supermarkets)
1 small yellow onion, chopped finely
2½ cups vegetable broth
2 tablespoons raisins
½ teaspoon curry powder
½ teaspoon turmeric powder (if you can find turmeric root, use 1 teaspoon minced)
½ teaspoon fresh ginger, minced
Pinch of sea salt and black pepper

Preparation
Preheat oven to 400°F. Pour the rice onto a baking sheet, spread out, and bake for 10 to 15 minutes or until the rice turns a golden brown. Stir around twice while toasting. Remove and set aside to cool. Spread the coconut flakes around on the same baking sheet and toast for 3 to 5 minutes, or until they start to brown. Be careful with these flakes because they toast fast and it's easy to over-toast

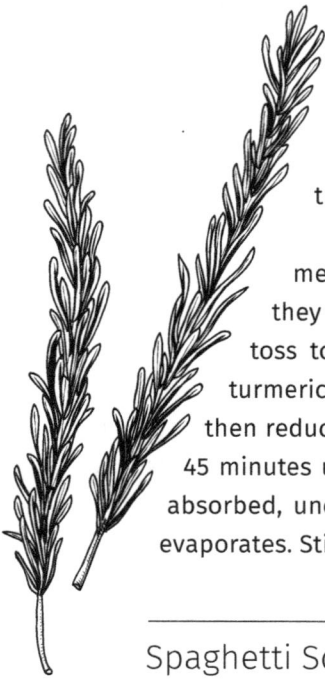

them. Remove from oven and set aside to cool. In a small saucepan, heat the butter on medium heat and sauté the chopped onions until they start to turn a light brown. Add the rice and toss to coat. Add the broth, raisins, curry powder, turmeric, ginger, sea salt, and pepper. Bring to a boil, then reduce the heat, cover, and simmer slowly for 40 to 45 minutes until the rice is tender. If the liquid isn't fully absorbed, uncover for a minute or two until excess liquid evaporates. Stir in the toasted coconut and serve.

Spaghetti Squash Spaghetti with Rustic Sauce

Ingredients
1 spaghetti squash, washed and halved
½ small yellow onion, diced
2 cloves garlic, minced
½ of a 6-oz can tomato paste
1 16-oz jar diced tomatoes
1 carrot, scrubbed and cut into thin rounds
¼ cup red bell pepper, diced
¼ cup green bell pepper, diced
⅛ cup yellow summer squash or zucchini, diced
1 medium stalk celery, diced (use the leaves of the celery chopped)

Spices
¼ teaspoon fresh rosemary, minced
½ teaspoon fresh oregano leaves, chopped
1 tablespoon flat-leaf parsley, chopped
1 tablespoon fresh basil, chopped
¼ teaspoon sea salt
Pinch of black pepper
Pinch of cayenne pepper

Preparation

Preheat oven to 350°F. Carefully cut the squash in half lengthwise and scoop out the seeds (you can wash and roast these for a nice snack). In a baking dish large enough to hold both halves of the squash, pour in ¼ inch of water. Place the squash halves cut side down in the dish. Cover the squash with foil and bake for 40 minutes.

To make the sauce, place a large, deep-sided pan over medium-low heat. Drizzle a small amount of coconut oil in the pan and add the onions. Sauté for 1 minute, and then add minced garlic and tomato paste. Sauté for 2 minutes, stirring frequently. This deepens the tomato paste's flavor. Add all the herbs and spices and stir for a few seconds, and then add diced tomatoes and carrots. Turn heat to a low simmer, cover, and let cook for 20 minutes.

After the sauce has cooked for 20 minutes, add the peppers, squash, and celery and simmer another 5 minutes. Turn off the heat and leave the saucepan covered.

When the squash is baked, carefully remove it from the baking pan using tongs. Over a large serving bowl, run a fork through the flesh of the squash from end to end. The squash will come out in long spaghetti-like strands.

Serve like regular spaghetti topped with tomato sauce.

Cold Soba Noodles with Lime Pesto Dressing

Ingredients

½ small English cucumber, deseeded
½ zucchini deseeded
2 tablespoons walnut halves
½ cup fresh basil leaves
½ cup fresh spinach, chopped
1 clove garlic, minced
2 tablespoons mellow white miso
2 tablespoons fresh ginger, minced

Zest and juice of 1 lime
Pinch of red pepper flakes
Vegetable broth
¼ teaspoon sea salt
Pinch of black pepper
1 pound of soba noodles
2 green onions, only the tops, chopped
¼ avocado, chopped
Fresh basil leaves, chopped

Preparation

Julienne the cucumber and zucchini. Toast the walnut halves in a pan over medium heat for 1 to 2 minutes, taking care not to burn or toast too long. Remove from the pan and chop finely.

To make the sauce, place the basil, spinach, minced garlic, miso, minced ginger, lime juice, red pepper flakes, and toasted walnuts in a blender and blend into a loose paste. If needed, loosen with a little vegetable broth. Add the lime zest and give it a quick pulse. Taste and add a little salt and pepper or a little more lime juice.

Cook the soba noodles per the instructions on the package. Drain well and rinse with cold water. Place them in a large serving bowl, pour the sauce over, and toss until noodles are thoroughly coated. Add the julienned vegetables and toss again.

Garnish with the chopped green onion, chopped avocado, and chopped basil. This is a great dish to serve with steamed broccoli or roasted asparagus.

Summertime Soba Pho

Ingredients for Broth/Sauce

32-oz carton vegetable broth (+ ½ cup)
2 whole star anise
1 teaspoon anise seeds
1 teaspoon Chinese five-spice powder

2 teaspoons fresh ginger, minced
2 cloves of garlic, smashed
Pinch of red pepper flakes (optional)
½ teaspoon sea salt
3 tablespoons Bragg Liquid Aminos or soy sauce
½ teaspoon fish sauce (optional for non-vegans)
1 tablespoon rice wine vinegar
½ teaspoon whole coriander seed, crushed
¼ cup dried mushrooms, shiitake
½ yellow onion, chopped
¼ cup baby portobello mushrooms, chopped

Main Dish Ingredients
½ red onion, sliced and pickled in rice wine vinegar (30 minutes)
One package of buckwheat or soba noodles
1 tablespoon extra-virgin olive oil
1 cup portobello mushrooms, cleaned and sliced
1 cup zucchini, halved and sliced
2 cups broccoli florets, washed and cut into bite-sized pieces
2 small bunches baby bok choy, washed, stems sliced and greens
chopped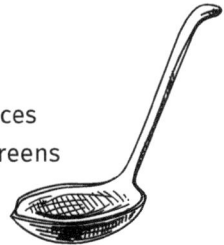
1 cup fresh basil leaf, washed and chiffonaded
¼ cup green onion, only the green tops, chopped
¼ cup cilantro, washed and chopped
1 cup of bean or pea sprouts
1 lime

Preparation
First, put the sliced red onion in a bowl along with enough red
wine vinegar to cover, and set aside. In a large saucepan add all
the broth/sauce ingredients and bring to near boil, reduce heat to
medium, and leave uncovered until this is reduced by half, about
30 to 40 minutes. You can speed up the reduction process by using
higher heat, but you need to stir often and make sure not to leave
the sauce unattended. Once the sauce is reduced you can cover

and let it stand for as long as you like, then strain it through a fine screen strainer. Take ½ of the reduction and set it aside. When you're ready to finish the dish, take the other ½ of the sauce and put it back in the saucepan and reduce to a semi-thick demi-glace (this should be the consistency of a light syrup). When you get this to the right consistency, remove from heat and cover.

Cook the noodles according to the instructions on the package. When the noodles are done, drain them. Place the noodles in the frying pan and pour the reserved first-reduction sauce over the noodles and toss until most of the liquid is absorbed. This should keep the noodles from sticking together while adding the flavors of the pho sauce. Here's a tip: if all the liquid is not absorbed, turn the heat to medium and allow the excess liquid to condense down, but you want a little of the sauce left because the noodles will continue to absorb it over time. Put the noodles into a large mixing or serving bowl and toss a couple of times while they cool, about 10 to 15 minutes; then they are ready to be served.

In a large, deep-sided frying pan over medium heat, add 1 tablespoon of extra-virgin olive oil, then add the mushrooms, zucchini, and broccoli florets and sauté for 2 minutes (do not overcook these as they should look fresh and have some crunch). Then add the bok choy and toss. Remove the veggies to a large bowl to stop the cooking process.

To serve, put ¼ of the cool noodles on a plate and place the sautéed vegetables, fresh basil, green onions, and the pickled red onions around the noodles.

Now drizzle some of the demi-glace over the top of the noodles and vegetables. Next, top with the chopped cilantro and the bean or pea sprouts. Add a couple wedges of fresh lime and serve. If you love the heat that many do when eating pho soup, you can put a few drops of Sriracha sauce on the noodles. Be careful; this dish is addictive. It takes some work to get the sauces right, but it is well worth the time.

You Won't Miss the Cheese Eggplant Lasagna

Ingredients
1 small to medium eggplant
1 yellow onion
1 package of whole wheat lasagna sheets
1 tablespoon tomato paste (Bionaturae Organic Tomato Paste if possible)
2 cloves garlic, minced
2 15-oz cans of tomato sauce
1 teaspoon dried Italian seasoning
1 teaspoon dried basil
1 teaspoon dried oregano
½ teaspoon sea salt
⅛ teaspoon black pepper
Pinch of red pepper flakes (optional)
2 celery stalks, diced
1 red bell pepper, diced
1 green bell pepper, diced
1 avocado, sliced
1 small can black olives, sliced

Tofu No-Cheese Mix
1 box firm tofu, drained and chopped
1 tablespoon sun-dried tomatoes, chopped
½ cup fresh basil, chopped
1 teaspoon capers, minced
2 teaspoons nutritional yeast
⅛ teaspoon garlic powder
⅛ teaspoon onion powder
⅛ teaspoon dried mustard powder
⅛ teaspoon sea salt
⅛ teaspoon black pepper
⅛ teaspoon turmeric
Pinch of paprika

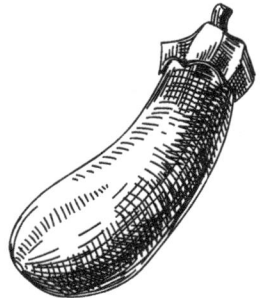

Preparation

Preheat the oven to 375° F. Slice the eggplant and onion into ¼-inch slices, brush a little olive oil on both sides, and salt and pepper lightly. Line a baking sheet with parchment paper and place the onion and eggplant slices on the baking sheet. Bake until they start to turn brown, about 15 to 20 minutes, making sure not to overbrown them, then turn them over and bake until the second side turns color, checking often. Remove from oven and set aside. Lower the oven temperature to 350° F. The roasted eggplant and onion add an incredible depth of flavor. Cook the lasagna sheets per instructions on the box. Do not use no-bake sheets because they are made from processed white flour.

Meanwhile, in a large pot, begin the tomato sauce by first adding the tomato paste and cooking it over medium heat for 2 minutes to deepen the flavor. Then add the minced garlic and stir into the tomato paste. Next add the tomato sauce and stir until well mixed. Add the Italian seasoning, dried basil, dried oregano, salt, pepper, and red pepper flakes. Cover and simmer for 20 minutes. In a small skillet sauté the celery and the red and green peppers for 2 minutes, seasoning with salt and pepper.

While the tomato sauce is cooking, begin the tofu no-cheese spread. In a food processor or a heavy-duty blender, add the tofu. Then add all the other ingredients and blend into a thick sauce. Almost paste-like is best. It does not need to be completely processed, but the sun-dried tomato and basil need to be broken down sufficiently. If the mix is too tight, add a little caper juice and the packing liquid from the sun-dried tomatoes or a little lemon juice.

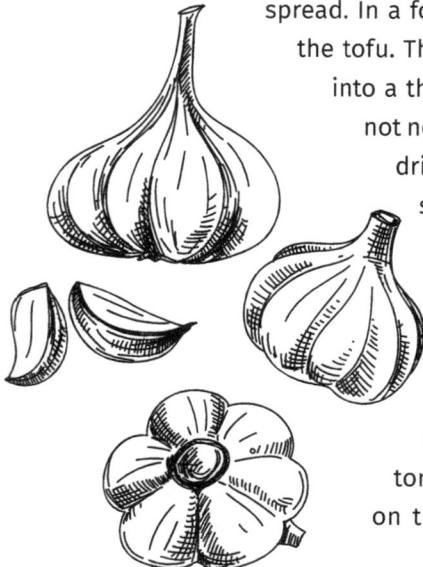

Building the lasagna

Coat a 9 × 13 baking pan with olive oil. Cover the bottom of the pan with ⅓ of the tomato sauce. Lay three of the lasagna sheets on the bottom of the pan. Then spread some of the tofu mix over them. Alternatively, you can use a spoon to scatter dollops of the mix over the lasagna sheets. Next, layer ½ of the onion and eggplant slices across the lasagna sheets and then top with ½ of the sautéed veggies and ½ of the sliced black olives, spreading them out evenly. Put down another layer of lasagna sheets and cover with ⅓ of the tomato sauce and repeat the procedure for the next layer. Finish by putting 3 more lasagna sheets down and cover with the remaining sauce. Cover with parchment paper and aluminum foil and put the baking pan into the oven on the middle rack and bake at 350°F for 30 minutes. When this is done, remove from the oven and let stand for 10 minutes.

To serve, cut into pieces and top with sliced avocado, some fresh chopped basil, and any of the remaining tofu mix.

For those with estrogen cancers, use soaked cashews in place of the tofu. Put 1½ cups of raw cashews in water, bring to boil for ten minutes, drain, and put in the blender in place of tofu. This is a big dish, so freeze what you don't eat for times when you are tired or do not have time to cook.

Mushroom Stroganoff with Caramelized Onions

Ingredients
1 yellow onion, sliced
1 cup plus 5 tablespoons vegetable broth
2 cups uncooked brown rice
2 cups assorted mushrooms (brown crimini, white button, shiitake, porcini), sliced
1 cup almond or rice milk
1 tablespoon vegan Worcestershire sauce
2 tablespoons Bragg Liquid Aminos or soy sauce
1 tablespoon balsamic vinegar
1 teaspoon garlic powder
¼ teaspoon turmeric
⅛ teaspoon paprika

⅛ teaspoon dried mustard powder
¼ teaspoon sea salt
⅛ teaspoon black pepper
3 tablespoons tofu sour cream
2 tablespoons cornstarch
⅛ cup parsley, chopped

Preparation

Cut the yellow onion in half lengthwise and thinly slice both halves. Heat a medium frying pan, add 2 tablespoons of vegetable broth, add the onions, and sauté on medium-low heat. Turn the onions every few minutes. You want a nice golden color, not burnt. This will take about 20 minutes. While the onions are caramelizing, cook the brown rice per package instructions. In a large skillet, add 3 tablespoons of vegetable broth and the sliced mushrooms. Cook over medium heat for 5 minutes. Add the caramelized onions, 1 cup vegetable broth, the almond milk, Worcestershire sauce, liquid aminos or soy sauce, balsamic vinegar, garlic powder, turmeric, paprika, dried mustard powder, and salt and pepper. Simmer for 15 minutes.

To finish this dish off, add the tofu sour cream and stir the mixture until well mixed. In a cup, combine cornstarch and 1 tablespoon of water and mix until the cornstarch completely dissolves. Turn the heat to medium and slowly add the cornstarch until the mixture thickens, making sure it's not too thick. When you get the desired thickness, turn the heat off and add the chopped parsley. Serve over the brown rice.

You can substitute a cashew sauce in place of the tofu sour cream by boiling a ½ cup of cashews for 10 minutes. Drain and put them into a blender along with a little water. Blend until you get a smooth, semi-loose mixture (add water as needed to get the thickness right). You will lose a little tanginess with this.

Basil Rosa Pasta

Ingredients

½ cup raw cashews, boiled
½ teaspoon fresh rosemary, minced
1 tablespoon extra-virgin olive oil
¼ yellow onion, diced finely
½ cup brown crimini mushrooms, sliced thinly
2 cloves garlic, minced
1 28-oz can crushed tomatoes
¼ teaspoon sea salt
Pinch of ground black pepper
2 teaspoons Truvia (sugar substitute)
1 package Barilla ProteinPLUS Linguini pasta
¼ cup black olives, sliced
½ cup fresh basil, chiffonaded

Preparation

Bring a large pot of water to a boil. At the same time bring 1½ cup of water to a boil in a small saucepan, reduce heat to low, and add the raw cashews. Simmer for 10 minutes and drain, saving the excess water. Put the boiled cashews in a blender along with a tablespoon of water and the minced rosemary. Blend on high speed until you get a nice smooth mixture, about 2 minutes. Add a little water if needed.

In a large saucepan, heat the olive oil over medium heat, then add the onion, mushrooms, and garlic and cook for 1 minute. Add the crushed tomatoes, sea salt, pepper, and Truvia. Turn heat to low, cover, and simmer for 15 minutes, stirring occasionally.

Add the linguini to the boiling water and cook according to package directions. While the pasta is cooking, stir cashew cream sauce into the tomato sauce and turn off the heat. Add the chopped olives and basil (reserving a little for garnish). When the pasta is done (slightly al dente), drain and put the pasta in a large serving bowl. Pour the finished sauce on the pasta and toss until well coated. Serve. (If you need to loosen the cashew sauce, add a little warm almond milk or rice milk and stir.)

Mediterranean Shell Pasta

Ingredients
½ small red onion, chopped roughly
1 tablespoon vegetable broth
½ cup red bell pepper, diced
⅓ cup celery, diced
½ cup zucchini, diced
⅓ cup marinated artichoke hearts, chopped
1 8-oz box of Ancient Harvest Quinoa pasta shells
1 cup spinach or chard, chopped
¼ cup fresh parsley, chopped
¼ cup Greek or kalamata olives, sliced
¼ cup black olives and green olives, sliced

Avocado Pesto Sauce
½ cup walnuts, chopped
2 cups fresh basil, chopped
½ avocado
2 cloves garlic, smashed
2 tablespoons fresh lemon juice
2 tablespoons extra-virgin olive oil
½ teaspoon sea salt
⅛ teaspoon ground black pepper
Pinch of cayenne pepper or pinch of red pepper flakes

Preparation
Bring a large pot of water to a boil. While water is boiling, prepare the pesto. First, place the walnuts in a small frying pan and toast them over medium heat,

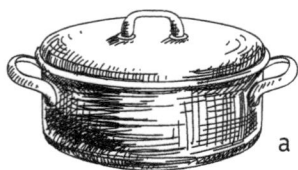

turning frequently until they just start to turn color. Remove from heat. Put all the ingredients for the pesto into a blender or food processor. Blend until the pesto is thick and smooth. If the mixture is too thick to blend, add some of the marinated artichoke juice, a little more lemon juice, or some more olive oil a little at a time to loosen the mix (if you use olive oil, take care not to overuse it). At the same time you are making the pesto, sauté the chopped red onion in the vegetable broth for 3 minutes, add the red peppers, celery, and zucchini and cook for another 2 minutes, tossing a couple times. Add the marinated artichoke hearts after you turn off the heat. Do not overcook this because you want the veggies to have some crunch to them. Set aside.

When the water for the pasta is ready, cook the shells per package instructions, drain, and save the pasta water. In a large serving bowl, put the chopped greens in first. Put the cooked pasta on top of the greens and let sit for a minute. Then dress with the pesto (use just enough to give the ingredients a nice coating). It should loosen and coat the pasta nicely. If more liquid is needed, carefully add a little of the pasta water, making sure not to dilute the sauce too much. Add the rest of the ingredients to the pasta and toss until well coated. At this point, you can use more pesto if needed or desired. To serve, put the pasta in a large pasta bowl and garnish with a little parsley and a few chopped walnuts for added crunch and flavor.

Open-Faced Italian Tofurky Sausage Sandwiches

Ingredients

1½ tablespoons extra-virgin olive oil

2 tablespoons of Bionaturae Organic Tomato Paste (comes in a 7-oz jar, love this stuff)

2 cloves garlic, minced

1 14.5-oz can tomato sauce

1 tablespoon dried oregano

1 teaspoon Italian dried seasoning

1 teaspoon fresh rosemary, minced

½ teaspoon caraway seed, crushed
½ teaspoon sea salt
⅛ teaspoon black pepper
Pinch of crushed red pepper flakes
3 Tofurky Italian sausage links, sliced into rounds
1 small red onion, halved and sliced
1 red bell pepper, julienned
1 green bell pepper, julienned
4 multigrain hoagie or sub-style buns, halved
1 tablespoon fresh basil, chopped

Preparation

Heat a medium-sized saucepan over medium heat and add 1 tablespoon extra-virgin olive oil, the tomato paste, and garlic and cook for 1 to 2 minutes, stirring so it doesn't burn. This will really add depth to the flavor. Add the tomato sauce, dried oregano, Italian seasoning, fresh rosemary, crushed caraway seeds (smash the seeds in a pestle or give them a quick burst in a spice grinder), sea salt, black pepper, and red pepper flakes. Turn the heat to simmer, cover, and cook for 15 minutes, stirring occasionally. This sauce should be a little thicker than pasta sauce, but not as thick as pizza sauce.

In a large skillet, heat ½ tablespoon of olive oil, then add the sliced Tofurky sausage over medium heat and brown until they show a dark brown color. Turn them until both sides are browned, then remove from pan and set aside. Add the onion slices and sauté for 2 minutes, stirring a couple times. Add the red and green bell peppers. Sprinkle on a little salt and pepper, and cook until they are soft but still maintain a little crunch, about 3 minutes. Turn off the heat.

To build the sandwich, put the bread halves cut side up under a broiler and brown. Place two halves on a plate, then spread 1 tablespoon of sauce on the bottom half and layer on first some of the sausage, then the onion and bell pepper mix. To finish off the sandwich, ladle some of the tomato sauce over the sandwich halves. Top the sandwiches with a little fresh basil and let sit for a minute so the sauce can soak into the bread. This isn't a finger food, so you will need a fork and knife. . . . YUM

Portobello Mushroom Burgers

Ingredients

1 tablespoon extra-virgin olive oil

2 tablespoons balsamic vinegar

1 tablespoon Dijon mustard

2 gloves garlic, minced

½ teaspoon vegan Worcestershire sauce

Salt and pepper

2 large portobello mushrooms, cleaned and destemmed

2 quarter-inch-thick red onion slices

1 red bell pepper, cut in half and roasted

2 large whole wheat burger buns

2 slices ripe tomato

½ cup arugula greens

Preparation

Preheat a grill on medium-high heat.

In a bowl, add the olive oil, balsamic vinegar, Dijon mustard, garlic, Worcestershire sauce, salt, and pepper and whisk until ingredients are well incorporated. Brush the mixture over the tops and bottoms of the mushrooms and let them sit for 10 minutes.

Place the basted mushrooms on the grill and cover them so the steam helps cook them through. When the first side is browned, turn and brown the other side, about 5 minutes per side. At the same time use a little of the basting sauce and brush the two slices of red onion and place them on the grill until they get a little brown. Turn and repeat.

To roast the pepper, turn a gas burner on high and place the pepper halves skin side down and cook until the shiny, waxy skin turns black and begins to blister. Once the skin is blackened, put the pepper halves in a plastic sandwich bag and close for 5 minutes. Then, remove them and peel off all the burnt skin.

To build the mushroom burger, toast the buns, spread some Dijon on the bun, put the grilled onion down first, then place the mushroom down, next the tomato slice and roasted red pepper, and finish off with some arugula leaves. Serve with oven-roasted sweet potato fries.

Veggie Black Bean Burritos with Susan's Guacamole and Pico de Gallo Salsa

Ingredients
2 cups uncooked brown rice
1 8-oz package Sweet Earth Traditional Seitan
2 cups cooked or 1 15-oz can black beans
½ cup water or vegetable broth
½ sweet yellow onion, finely diced
2 avocados
1 small red onion, sliced
1 ripe tomato, diced
½ cup cilantro, chopped finely
2½ limes
1 jalapeño pepper
1 package whole wheat flour tortillas, large or burrito sized
1 green bell pepper, julienned
½ cup corn, seasoned with lime and chili powder
⅛ cup green onion tops, chopped

Spices
1½ (+) teaspoon cumin
1 (+) teaspoon chili powder
⅛ (+) teaspoon smoked paprika
1 (+) teaspoon garlic powder

½ teaspoon onion powder
Pinch of cayenne pepper
½ teaspoon Mexican oregano
¼ teaspoon Louisiana Hot Sauce
Sea salt
Black pepper

Preparation

Make the brown rice. In this recipe I make more rice than I need for the meal because having extra rice is always handy. Next, separate the seitan sheets (3 to 4 depending on the thickness of the sheets), and lay them out on a piece of wax paper. To get a taco meat flavor, sprinkle some cumin, chili powder, smoked paprika, garlic powder, onion powder, and a little cayenne pepper on both sides, then stack the seasoned sheets on top of one another and allow them to rest and absorb the flavors of the spices (these spices are in addition to the ones listed above). To make the black beans, you can either make your own or use one 15-ounce can, drained and washed. Put the cooked beans in a medium saucepan, and add ½ cup water or vegetable broth. Add ¼ cup of finely diced sweet yellow onion, cumin, chili powder, garlic powder, onion powder, smoked paprika, and a pinch of cayenne pepper. Simmer on low heat for 15 minutes, then turn off the heat and set aside.

Susan's Guacamole

Start by marinating 1 tablespoon of the finely diced onion in a bowl with the juice of ½ a lime and the hot sauce and set aside. Dice the avocados into small cubes and put them into a medium-sized mixing bowl. Add ⅛ cup finely chopped cilantro and salt and pepper and the marinated onion. Mix gently and set aside.

Pico de Gallo Salsa

Dice 1 ripe tomato and put in a small mixing bowl. Add 2 tablespoons of very finely diced sweet yellow onion, 1 teaspoon finely minced jalapeño pepper, ¼ cup finely chopped cilantro, the juice of 1 small lime, and a pinch of salt and black pepper. Set aside.

When the rice is done, separate it into halves, saving one half for another day. Take the other half and add ¼ cup finely chopped cilantro, chopped green onion tops, the Mexican oregano, juice of ½ small lime, ¼ teaspoon cumin, a pinch of salt, and black pepper, mixing the rice thoroughly.

In a medium-sized skillet over medium heat, add the sliced red onion and sauté for 4 to 5 minutes, tossing to make sure they don't burn. Add the green bell peppers and cook for another 3 minutes. Lightly salt and pepper and squeeze a little lime juice over the mixture, then remove from the pan. To make the seitan, cut into ¼-inch strips. In the skillet, still over medium heat, add the seitan strips and brown them, tossing a couple times. Set aside.

To soften the tortillas, place them in between a couple of damp dish towels and put them in the microwave for 45 seconds or so. They should be pliable. To make the burritos, heat a large skillet over low heat. Place a tortilla in the skillet and warm it up so it's pliable. Remove from the pan and place on a cutting board. Using a slotted spoon to make sure the beans are drained, spread out a layer of the black beans over the burrito. Next put on a few of the seitan strips, but not too many. Now, spread out about 2 tablespoons of the rice mixture and add a layer of grilled onions and green bell peppers and 1 tablespoon of the seasoned corn (at this point you can also add a tablespoon of tofu sour cream if you like). Now, take the tortilla and pull the short side all the way over the filling, fold the sides in, and then roll up the tortilla. Place in the heated pan seam side down and repeat, making as many burritos as you need.

To serve, place two burritos on a plate, and top them with the pico de gallo and one tablespoon of Susan's guacamole per burrito. Serve with some of the extra black beans and rice on the side. Garnish with a little cilantro and a spritz of lime juice.

Seitan is made from whole wheat, not soy, and can be found at many supermarkets such as Whole Foods, Mother's, Trader Joe's, Sprouts, or other markets that carry alternative vegan-type foods. It comes in several brands and flavors. Always read the label because some flavored varieties have added sugar, a no-no for cancer patients.

Seitan Fajitas

Ingredients
1 tablespoon extra-virgin olive oil
1 8-oz package seitan, sliced into thin strips
1 small red onion, sliced
2 tablespoons vegetable broth
2 tablespoons Bragg Liquid Aminos or soy sauce
3 cloves garlic, minced
½ teaspoon fresh ginger, minced
1 teaspoon paprika (preferably smoked)
1 teaspoon cumin powder
½ teaspoon coriander powder
2 teaspoons chili powder
Pinch of cayenne pepper
1 red bell pepper, julienned
1 green bell pepper, julienned
2 limes
⅓ cup cilantro, chopped
1 package whole wheat tortillas
1 avocado, peeled, deseeded, and sliced
Tofutti Better Than Sour Cream (optional)
Salsa (like Trader Joe's Salsa Autentica or Pace)

Preparation
Heat the olive oil on medium heat in a large skillet and add the seitan strips. Brown the strips for 2 minutes, then turn to brown the other side. Add the onion and cook for 4 minutes. Then, add the broth and liquid aminos or soy sauce along with the garlic, ginger, paprika, cumin powder, coriander powder, chili powder, and a small pinch of cayenne pepper. Lower the heat to medium-low and sauté for 2 minutes. Add the red and green peppers and sauté for another 2 to 3 minutes (the peppers should have a little crunch

to them), toss a couple times, then add the juice of the limes and the chopped cilantro and toss again. Sauté until the liquid has been absorbed and evaporated. Turn off the heat.

Steam the tortillas and add the filling. Top with a couple avocado slices, salsa, and a squeeze of lime. There is a lot of spice in this dish and it will look like too much, but it's not; they add so much flavor that I'm sure this will become one of your favorites. I also like to spread out a tablespoon of Tofutti Better Than Sour Cream on the tortillas before adding the seitan and peppers.

Mexican Black Bean Lasagna with Avocado and Cilantro

Ingredients
1 cup corn kernels
1 lime
Pinch of chili powder
4 cups mashed homemade black beans or 4 cups vegetarian refried black beans
1 cup green onions, chopped
½ cup black olives, sliced
¼ cup Spanish green olives, sliced
1 7-oz can Ortega Diced Green Chiles
1 teaspoon jalapeño, deseeded and minced
1 tablespoon olive oil
10 to 12 corn tortillas
½ cup cilantro, chopped
1 large avocado
1 fresh tomato, diced

Sauce
2 8-oz cans tomato sauce
3 cups water
¼ cup cornstarch

2 tablespoons chili powder
½ teaspoon onion powder
½ teaspoon garlic powder
½ teaspoon turmeric
⅛ teaspoon smoked paprika
¼ teaspoon ground cumin

Sauce preparation

In a large saucepan, add all the sauce ingredients and whisk thoroughly. Turn the heat to medium and cook, whisking occasionally until the sauce thickens, approximately 5 minutes. Season, adding salt or chili powder to desired taste. Set aside.

Chili-lime corn preparation

Make the chili-lime corn by placing the corn kernels into a frying pan over medium heat. Add ½ of the lime juice and shake on some chili powder. Set aside.

Assembling the dish

Preheat oven to 350°F. In a large mixing bowl combine the beans (warm them beforehand), green onions (reserve ⅛ cup), black and green olives, chili-lime corn kernels, diced green chiles, and minced jalapeños and mix thoroughly. Now, lightly coat a 9 ×13 baking pan with olive oil and spread 1 cup of the sauce on the bottom. Put down 3 to 4 tortillas or as many as needed to cover the baking dish. Spread half of the bean mixture over the tortillas. Cover the bean mix with another layer of tortillas and top with the rest of the bean mix. Cover the bean mix with 3 to 4 more tortillas and pour the remaining sauce over them. Take ⅛ cup of the chopped green onion tops and ¼ cup chopped cilantro and spread evenly over the sauce. Cover with parchment paper and then cover the paper with aluminum foil, making sure to crimp the edges over the baking dish. Put in the oven and cook for 45 minutes.

Remove from the oven and let rest for 15

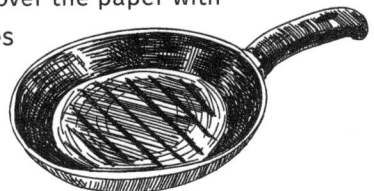

minutes. While waiting for this to set, make an avocado topping. Scoop the avocado flesh into a dish, mashing it with a fork until most of the lumps are gone, then add the remaining chopped cilantro, the juice of ¼ of a lime, and a little salt and pepper to taste and mix again. To serve, carefully remove the foil and parchment paper, cut into serving sizes, top with the avocado mix and diced tomatoes.

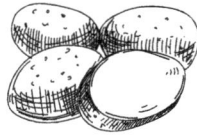

Side Dishes

You can make a lot of dishes as sides. Baked sweet potatoes and russet potatoes, brown rice dishes with herbs and spices added. Try Old World grains such as bulgur, barley, faro, and sorghum. They haven't yet been genetically engineered, and most are very high in protein. You can make lots of delicious dishes with them, and people will love them because most likely they haven't eaten these grains.

Pineapple Ginger Quinoa

Ingredients
1 cup rainbow quinoa
1 teaspoon coconut oil or extra-virgin olive oil
¼ cup red onion, chopped finely
¼ pineapple, chopped
1 clove garlic, minced finely
1 tablespoon fresh ginger root, minced
Zest and juice of ½ lemon
Pinch of cayenne pepper
1 tablespoon pineapple juice
⅓ cup mint leaves, chopped

Preparation
Make the quinoa per package instructions.
While the quinoa is cooking, prep all the other ingredients and heat a small nonstick pan over medium-low heat. Add the coconut oil, red onion, and pineapple and sauté for 2 minutes. Add garlic, ginger root, lemon zest, lemon juice, cayenne pepper, and pineapple juice and sauté for 1 minute longer, then remove from the heat.

When the quinoa is finished cooking, uncover and fluff it with a fork, and let it stand for a few minutes. The quinoa should look like fluffy rice when ready. When it reaches that point, pour the sauce from the pan into the quinoa and mix well. Mix in the mint leaves and serve.

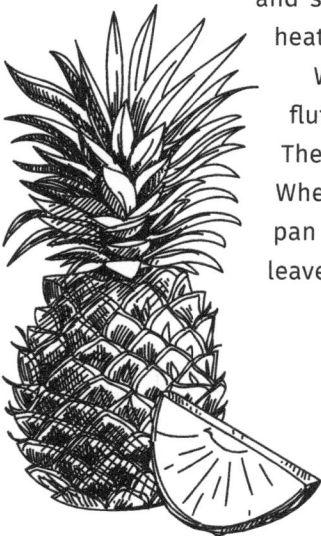

Spicy Roasted Red Yam Rounds

Ingredients
1 lime
1 large red yam (try to find one with a regular shape and uniform thickness along its length)
2 teaspoons extra-virgin olive oil

Spices
Cumin
Chili powder
Smoked paprika
Black pepper
Sea salt

Preparation
Preheat oven to 375° F. Quarter the lime. Wash the yam thoroughly, but do not peel it. Dry the yam and cut into round ¼-inch-thick slices; slice it a little thicker if you want, but not thinner. Put the slices into a large mixing bowl and toss with the olive oil to coat the yam rounds. Line a baking sheet with parchment paper or foil and place the rounds on the sheet.

Sprinkle on the salt, black pepper, and cumin first. Then, turn the yam rounds over and sprinkle on the chili powder and smoked paprika and a little extra sea salt.

Place the baking sheet in the oven for 20 minutes, checking at 10 and 15 minutes to make sure the yams aren't burning. When you see them start to turn color, turn them over, roast for 5 minutes, and then check both sides. They should be uniformly light brown.

When they are finished roasting, take them out of the oven and squeeze lime juice on each piece, allowing the juice to soak in.

These are so good. Eat them hot as a snack or serve as a side dish. I also make roasted chickpeas just like this with the same spices.

I toast the chickpeas until they are crunchy, add a little lime juice, and then snack on them instead of nuts.

Loco Crazy Good Hummus

Ingredients

1 15-oz can chickpeas (garbanzo beans), drained and rinsed
or ½ cup dry, then cooked
¼ (+) cup fresh lemon juice
¼ cup tahini
2 tablespoons extra-virgin olive oil
½ teaspoon garlic powder
⅛ teaspoon onion powder
½ teaspoon ground cumin
½ teaspoon paprika
¼ teaspoon turmeric powder
⅛ teaspoon chili powder
½ teaspoon sea salt
⅛ teaspoon ground black pepper
3 to 4 tablespoons El Pato Tomato Sauce with or without Jalapeño
(hot Mexican tomato sauce)

Preparation

First, I like to make my own chickpeas, but it takes time, so for convenience use the canned variety. Here is a good tip: after you rinse the chickpeas, take the thin translucent shell off of them. This will take 10 minutes, but it's worth the time because you get a smoother hummus.

In a food processor, add the fresh lemon juice and tahini and process for 1 minute. Stop and scrape down the sides and process for another 30 seconds. This will whip the tahini and give your finished hummus a great smoothness.

Add the extra-virgin olive oil, garlic powder, onion powder, cumin, paprika, turmeric, chili powder, sea salt, and black pepper and process for 1 minute, stop and scrape down the sides, and process for 30 seconds.

Add ½ of the rinsed and shelled chickpeas and process for 1 minute, scrape down the sides, and add the rest of the chickpeas, process for two minutes, scrape down the sides again, then add 3 to 4 tablespoons of El Pato Tomato Sauce and process for another minute.

Taste and re-season the hummus if you want, but this is flavor-packed the way it is

Tabbouleh Salad

Ingredients
¼ cup dry 10-minute bulgur
½ cup water
1 cup parsley, chopped
¼ cup mint, chopped
3 to 5 fresh ripe tomatoes, deseeded and diced
1 small yellow onion, diced finely
1 lemon, juiced
2 teaspoons extra-virgin olive oil
1 teaspoon garlic powder
⅛ teaspoon sea salt
¼ cup English cucumber, diced

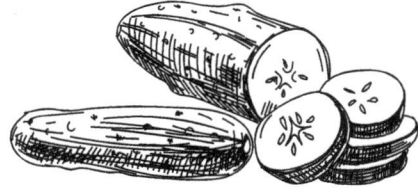

Preparation
Prepare the quick-cooking bulgur per package instructions. If you can't find quick-cooking bulgur, use Bob's Red Mill Bulgur and prepare per package instructions. In a large mixing bowl, combine the parsley, mint, tomatoes, onion, cucumber, lemon juice, olive oil, garlic powder, and salt, mix well, and let rest for 30 minutes to incorporate the flavors. I love this recipe and it keeps very well when refrigerated, so I often double or triple it.

Oven-Baked Sweet Potato Cinnamon Fries

Ingredients

1 medium-sized sweet potato

1 tablespoon extra-virgin olive oil

3 teaspoons ground cinnamon

1 teaspoon Cajun spice

½ teaspoon sea salt

1 teaspoon Truvia sweetener

Preparation

Preheat the oven to 375° F. Cut the sweet potato into ¼-inch slabs, then cut again into ¼-inch slices (french-fry style). Put the cut sweet potato fries into a large mixing bowl and add the olive oil and toss, coating the potatoes thoroughly. Sprinkle the spices over the coated fries and toss until the spices are evenly distributed. Then, put some parchment paper or aluminum foil over a baking sheet, and spread the sweet potatoes fries over the sheet in a single layer. Bake in the oven for 15 to 20 minutes, checking them a couple times. When the down side of the fries becomes a golden brown, turn them over and bake for another 5 minutes. They will brown faster after they are turned. When the fries are all nice and golden, take them out of the oven and serve. These can be used as a snack as well as part of a meal

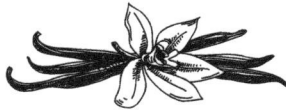

Desserts

Flourless Chocolate Chocolate Chip Walnut Cookies

Makes 20–25 small cookies

Ingredients

2 flax eggs: 2 tablespoons ground flax + 6 tablespoons water (Bob's Red Mill Golden Ground Flax is inexpensive)

1 cup organic almond butter

¼ cup raw cacao powder (or Hershey's Cocoa Natural Unsweetened powder)

1 cup stevia-sweetened Lilly's dark chocolate chips

½ cup organic walnuts, chopped

½ teaspoon baking soda

¼ teaspoon pink Himalayan salt or sea salt

Preparation

Preheat the oven to 350°F. Prepare the flax eggs: in a small bowl, whisk the ground flaxseed and water and set aside.

If the almond butter has been refrigerated, warm it to room temperature. In a medium-sized bowl, add the ingredients (the order isn't important) and the flax eggs and stir until well combined. Make sure to get all the dry ingredients on the bottom of the bowl mixed in.

For drop cookies: drop a spoonful at a time onto your baking pan. For rounder, traditional cookies: drop a spoonful at a time onto your baking pan, then pat the drops down lightly with your fingertips to flatten them slightly, then use your fingertips to pat the edges to smooth them out.

Bake for 10 minutes. Cool completely before removing from the baking pan, then refrigerate (very important).

Chocolate Nut and Fruit Energy Bars

Ingredients

1⅓ cups uncooked rolled oats

1 cup whole wheat flour

¼ cup dried cranberries

¼ cup dried tart red cherries

¼ cup dried prunes, chopped

½ cup chopped nuts: almonds, peanuts, pistachios

¼ cup walnuts, chopped

¼ cup sunflower seeds

¼ cup unsweetened cocoa powder

¼ cup vegan chocolate protein powder (not soy protein based)

¼ cup sugar-free chocolate chips or 85% chocolate bar chopped up

1 teaspoon baking powder

½ teaspoon baking soda

½ teaspoon ginger powder

1 teaspoon sea salt

¾ cup natural peanut or almond butter

¼ cup almond milk

1 tablespoon agave

¼ cup coconut sugar

1 teaspoon cinnamon

1 teaspoon vanilla extract

2 flax eggs (2 tablespoons of ground flaxseed + 6 tablespoons water mixed together)

Preparation

Preheat oven to 375° F. Lightly coat a 9 × 13 pan with coconut oil or an oil spray used judiciously.

In a large mixing bowl, add all the dry ingredients. Make sure the chopped nuts and dried fruit pieces aren't too big. Toss the mixture and set aside.

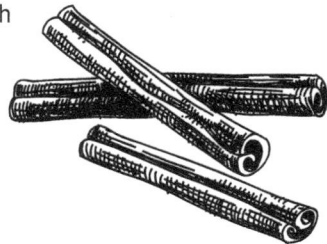

Add the peanut or almond butter to a saucepan over low heat, then add the almond milk and stir. Add the agave, coconut sugar, cinnamon, vanilla extract, and flax eggs. Stir until well mixed. The mixture should be semi-loose, but thicker than cake batter.

Stir in the mixture with the dry ingredients using a wooden spoon. Make sure all the dry ingredients get mixed with the wet. If the mixture is too thick, add more almond milk to loosen it up. The final consistency should be that of cookie dough.

With a rubber spatula, spread the mixture evenly in the pan. Then with your hand on the spatula end, press down on the mix to ensure it covers the pan.

Bake for 11 to 13 minutes, taking care not to overbake. Remove pan and allow to cool completely before cutting.

Epilogue

THIS MORNING (June 17, 2015) I checked my email and saw a notification of a new entry in Drew Hilliard's journal. Reluctantly—because for the past couple of weeks the news has been as bad as it could get—I logged in to read it.

Then, I got up, walked over to Susan, took her hand, and gently pulled her to her feet and put my arms around her. I told her I had just read Drew's latest entry.

"I have to make this book good." Then I broke down and cried.

"Just make it as good as you can. You can't always change the way people live."

I held her even tighter and said, "I don't want to go through that with you." And then really let the tears go.

I am incredibly sad to say that Drew passed away at 5:17 p.m. on Monday, June 15, 2015. We knew this was coming, yet it still really hit both of us hard because we were deeply invested in Drew's fight with his cancer.

He inspired us for a number of reasons. The first time was when he sent us his awesome photo and message. Then we found out he too was fighting cancer and was winning the fight and was also writing an online journal. When I read his story I was amazed at how much work he did studying the medicines he was being treated with and the other treatment options that were available to him.

Next it was the selfless work he did to raise money for the fight against cancer. When his doctors found one tiny spot in his lung in 2013, two years after he thought he beat cancer, it was a cause for concern. He got the terrible news some months later that his cancer was back, and again we marveled at how he went about his fight by seeking out the top doctors who specialized in the rare cancer he had and by exploring every treatment option available to him.

But, sadly, this time his cancer was too smart and too aggressive. And this past week we again were inspired by how graciously and eloquently he went about the last days of his young life.

Susan and I owe a great deal to Drew. We will never forget this young Navy lieutenant. We never met Drew, but we know him and what kind of man he was. I think he lived as good as he could, and he did his best.

When I talk to young people about business and about life, I tell them their journey down life's road will have many surprises along the way. And I tell them not to be afraid to step over the white lines marking the edges of the road and to walk out into the unknown, take chances, and prepare to be amazed and bruised and bloodied. I tell them to enjoy what they can and appreciate the rest. I tell them to never give up even when things look hopeless because it's then that you learn who you are and what is important in life, and sometimes you see miracles unfold right before your eyes.

As Susan traveled her road, she picked up an unwanted passenger. This uninvited hitchhiker has forever altered the way she lives. And it has changed where I am headed in my journey. When we found out she was stage 4 and her cancer could not be cured, I decided I would do everything I could to help her, and later I felt an overwhelming desire to help others. It became my mission to fight her cancer and then cancer in general.

The decision to write this book was based on the feedback I got from hundreds of folks who heard her story and how we put up our fight.

Today is so bittersweet for us. On one hand, hearing about Drew has shaken us to the core. On the other hand, Susan is now in remission, and so far she is winning her battle. Even though she has been called a miracle girl, we have again been reminded that the war is a long way from being over. We are not proclaiming victory here because with a cancer diagnosis there is no final victory.

However, I don't think there is any final defeat either. For the moment, we are relieved and grateful that Susan is cancer free. We pray for a long future together filled with peace. It took a lot of hard work to get here and the help of hundreds of people. She found out who her friends are, and they are many, and we grew closer together. She also found an inner strength she didn't know she had.

♻

Last fall I took a couple of elective classes that I didn't need for the degree in nutrition I'm working toward. I had to make a tough decision: finish the classes or write this book. Susan told me to do the book; the classes could wait, she said. She felt like the book was important because it could help so many people who are fighting cancer and help prevent it.

So, I changed course, and in doing so I am fulfilling the promise I made to her and to others and the promise I made to myself that I would help as many people as I could to live life without going through what Susan has or, God forbid, what Drew did.

Cancer never quits; it learns and grows stronger and more virulent. So, we can't quit either, and we have to keep learning how to fight this disease because that will make us stronger, too.

We are now almost four years removed from the date of Susan's diagnosis and nearly a year from the last time I wrote in our journal. I think about her journey every single day, and most of those days I tell her story to a stranger. Not one of them wasn't moved or impressed.

I have one advantage over everyone because I see Susan every day. I see how hard she fights and how dedicated she is to sticking to the plan and trusting that this was and is the right course of action. I see firsthand her toughness and strength, I've witnessed her grace in the darkest of times, and I feel her compassion for every living thing. I've seen and heard from people who have been changed by her. This makes me realize how lucky I am, and I thank God that she is my wife.

Baby, I hope this book is good enough.

Jessica Jazz
2000–2015
We lost Jessica Jazz at 4:05 p.m. on July 27, 2015. Jessie was fifteen and a half years old and spent all but twelve weeks of her life with us. Jessie was Susan's best friend, and the bond between them was remarkable.

Susan rescued Jessie from a pet store, and in turn Jessie repaid Susan by saving her life when she told us Susan had cancer. For the last several weeks of her life, it was evident the end was near for Jessie. She was in a lot of pain and had stopped eating. She could no longer get up on her own or stand for very long without someone holding her up. Sunday we knew we couldn't watch her suffer any longer and made the decision to put her to sleep.

In Jessie's last moments, Susan leaned down and hugged her and said, "I love you, puppy dog." And she did with all her heart.

Jessica Jazz came to us from a Kansas puppy mill. She filled our lives with happiness and love. She will always hold a special place in all our hearts.

Mick
2004–2015
My dog, Mick, went to heaven to be reunited with Jessie on August 11, just fifteen days after Jessie's passing. Mick had a very aggressive cancer that ended his life far too soon. He fought his cancer much like Susan fought hers. He never complained and he never let his pain get him down.

Mick was my constant companion, and he was my friend and confidant in the truest sense, but he also was everyone's friend. His nickname was Tigger because that's who he acted like. He bounced and flounced and he ran with great enthusiasm. Mick lived life with pure joy, and in doing so he brought joy to all of us. He always had a smile on his face, even as he drew his last breath.

The passing of Jessie and Mick has left huge holes in our lives. But these two also left us with many irreplaceable memories.

Acknowledgments

IN MY WILDEST dreams I never thought I would write a book. For starters, English was never my favorite subject in school, that is, until I went back to college in 2009. I can't spell and I am dyslexic, so writing is a slow process for me. But I have lived long enough to know that anything is possible and miracles can happen. On rare occasions there is a convergence of events that opens up possibilities and delivers miracles.

When I went back to college, my goal was to get a master's degree in economics so I could teach. I had to retake my academic writing classes. I was not thrilled about that and tried to get out of taking them, but my requests were denied.

My first writing professor was Michael Lathrop, and we had an instant connection because he was from Eugene, Oregon, just eighty miles from where I grew up. His teaching style was perfect for me, so I actually had fun learning how to write. Because his class was a beginning writing class, I had to spend twenty-four hours in a writing lab, and that is where it all got started for me.

The professor who reviewed all my work and helped me was Brenda Borron. She was the first one to see potential in me and helped more than her job required. I can't tell you how many hours I spent in her office talking about writing and life in general. She has since become one of my dear friends and biggest cheerleaders.

Then I met Professor Julie Evans, who taught me the fundamentals and how to organize and write academic essays. Julie's class was tough, and she was demanding. Her class is the only writing class that I did not get an A in, and I've never been prouder of a B than the one I earned from her.

My next class is where everything changed because I met one of the most influential people in my life, Professor Shaina Trapedo. Shaina had us all keep journals as part of her class. We could write about anything. My journal ended up being a running conversation with Shaina on topics that were personal to me. She guided me, counseled me, and most of all she inspired me to write every day and not to fear writing down my thoughts and sharing them with others.

After I finished my academic writing classes, Professor Borron convinced me to take creative writing classes. That is when I met Marie Connors, whom I am delighted to count as a friend. If I needed extra help, she was always happy to review my work in her spare time, and she would read pieces I had written for other classes and offer her opinions.

Wendy Esteras taught me how to write poetry—well, at least to try to write it. She was another professor who took the time to help me whenever I needed it. Then I took a creative writing workshop class taught by a very special woman, Professor Lisa Alvarez. Lisa had to endure my writing for three years. I can't thank her enough for all the help she has given me. In fact, Professor Alvarez was the one who helped me start my blog.

I can honestly say these professors changed my life forever because of the confidence and knowledge they gave me. They are the ones who made it possible for me to write this book.

Right after Susan was diagnosed with cancer and I knew diet was going to be a part of how we would attack her disease, I called John Liviakis. John is the founder and CEO of Liviakis Financial Communications, and that's where I first came into contact with him. Later, I went to work for him, and he became a mentor. John is one of the smartest people I have ever meet. He is also a strong advocate for eating a vegan diet. His has owned vegan restaurants and knows more about food and its effects on health than most dietitians. The information he provided was instrumental in how I developed our dietary plan.

Others who have made this book possible are David Gomez, who I worked for and who then became my partner in Premier Capital. Susan was diagnosed right after we started our company, and David was a big help to us financially and made sure I had all the time I needed to care for Susan.

In 2013, I had to take on a part-time job. I called Lundun Morgan. I had worked for his home improvement company for a short time a few years earlier, and he was kind enough to hire me and let me work a limited schedule. One day while I was driving home, Julie, his wife, called me and asked if I would come to work full time for them. I told her that might be hard because Susan was my highest priority and if she needed me I had to be there for her. I told Julie I was going to college, which was also a priority. She told me not to worry and that she would work it out. I said okay.

Lundun and Julie made it possible for me to care for Susan, go to college full time, and still make a living. They have always given me the time I needed to accomplish everything I wanted to do, including writing this book. I don't know how many people can say they love who they work for, but I do. I talk to Julie all the time, and she constantly encourages me and lifts my spirits when they need a little boost.

I want to thank Dr. Simon Davies for writing the foreword for this book. And for taking the time to counsel me on diet and nutrition. He taught me so much, and I am forever grateful and indebted to him.

When I started writing the book, I knew I would need a good editor. I was not yet part of the writing community and didn't really know where to look, so I did Internet searches. I also asked a good friend, Steve Bjorkman, a widely published author, about what to look for in an editor and if he had any tips. One thing he told me was be careful because it's easy to make a mistake. That was good advice. After weeks of searching and background checks, I had a long list of editors. I decided I wanted to meet with six of them to discuss this project. Then I narrowed it down to three, and Susan and I met with them one last time. One editor, Naomi Long Eagleson, and her company, The Artful Editor, stood out because she presented us with a complete plan in which everything was laid out for us, and she was so professional. We wanted to entrust our story to her, but I didn't know if I could afford someone of her caliber. Susan and I knew if we were going to do this, we had to do it right because we both believed this was an important project. If Naomi was willing to take on our book, we would find a way to make it happen. Working with Naomi has been such an incredible experience, and she has been a blessing.

I also want to thank Susan's coworkers, Francesca Capella Smith, Lisa Alvarez, Jesus Rodriquez, and Kim Maffioli, for everything they have done for Susan.

Susan and I are extremely blessed with great parents, Martin and Ann Schreffler and Willis and Sandra Weaver. Their support, spiritual and financial, for Susan provided more than words can describe. Our children, Joshua and Nicole, have been instrumental in helping us implement our strategy, and without their help Susan's fight would have been so much harder.

Lastly, I want to thank my friend Peter Gerrard, who was instrumental in the production of our promotional video and photographs, and provided us with wise counsel. Plus I need to thank one of my oldest friends, Kathy Markham Aalto, who has helped to promote this book and has given me great advice. And thanks also to everyone who contributed to our Kickstarter campaign. You know who you are.

I am not sure how many people witness true miracles. I can now count myself among those who have. I am privileged and honored to have been by Susan's side as she courageously battled one of the biggest killers in the world, with all the odds stacked against her, and to see her gain the upper hand. I am in awe of how she has waged that battle.

I think back to what I've asked of God in my prayers. I remember the conversation I had with him that day on my walk about why I was put on earth and how I thought I was supposed to do something important. He told me to take stock of my life and to look at what was going on around me. He told me to think about it. In the past four years, I've done a lot of that.

Through this reflection I realized that I have met the right people at the right time who have opened new possibilities for me. The miracle was provided by Susan. Maybe my purpose is to write her story and remind people that with enough work and faith the possibilities are limitless and miracles do happen. And as Susan says . . .

Just don't give up.

About the Author

JEFFERY WEAVER was born in Myrtle Creek, Oregon in 1949. He eventually transitioned from college track-and-field star to business owner, working in the timber, communications, and financial services industries. Though a lifelong student of economics, he gained an interest in nutrition as the result of his wife's cancer diagnosis. Jeff lives in Brea, California with his wife, Susan. They have two children, Joshua and Nicole, and two Australian Shepherds, Cooper and Bounce.

More information can be found at www.jefferyweaver.com.

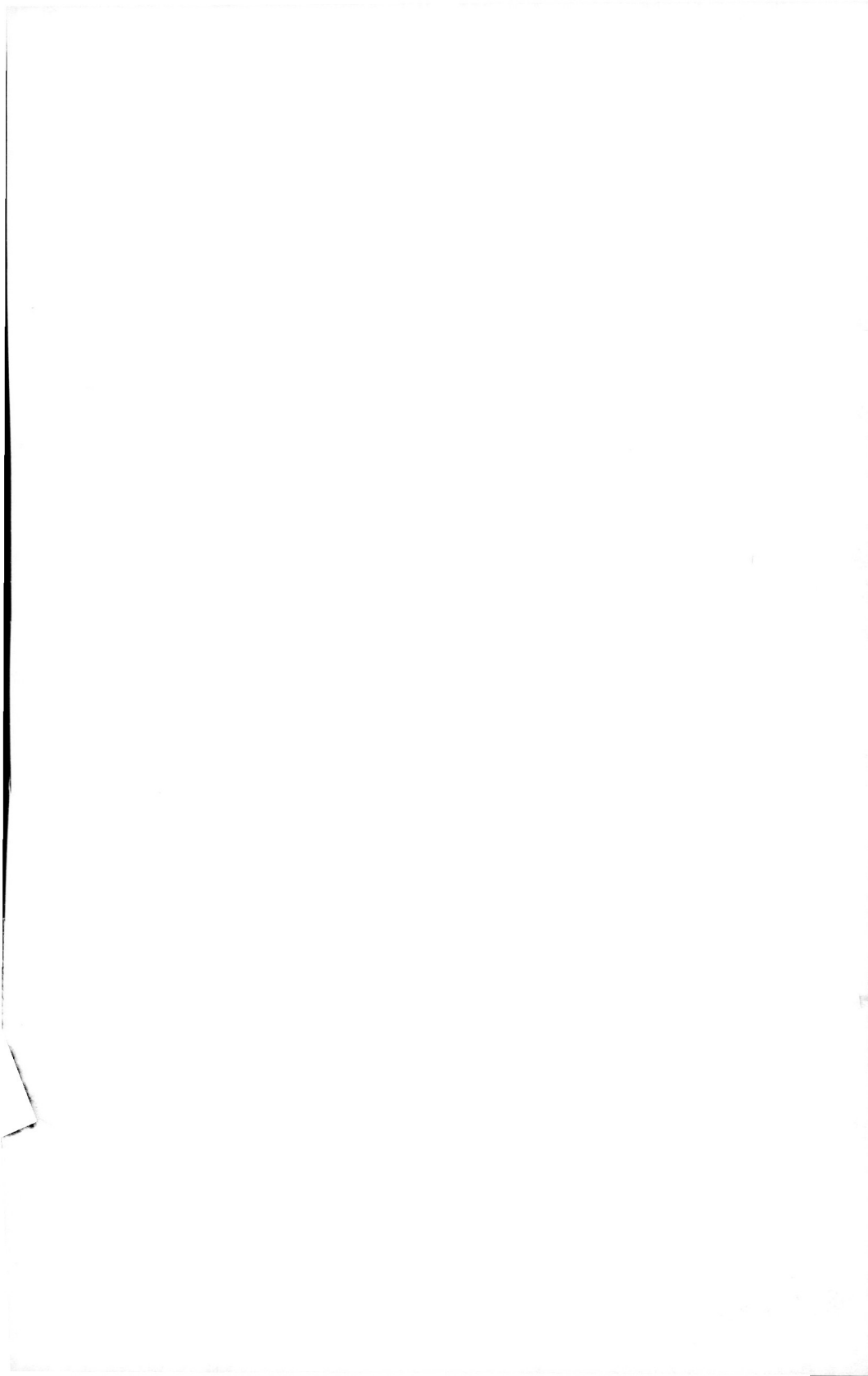

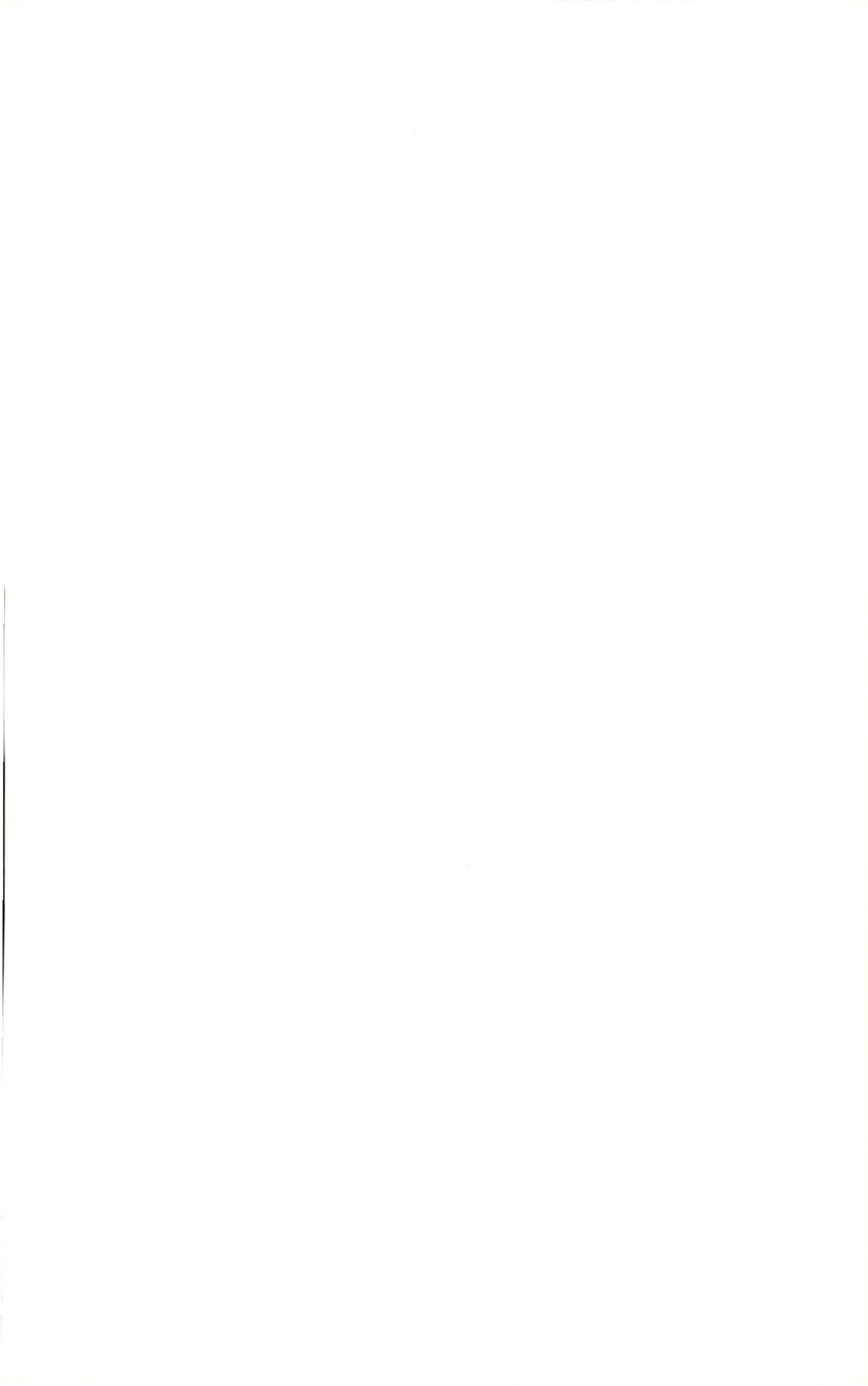